STP 1305

Safety in American Football

Earl F. Hoerner, editor

ASTM Publication Code Number (PCN):
04-013050-47

ASTM
100 Barr Harbor Drive
West Conshohocken, PA 19428-2959
Printed in the U.S.A.

Library of Congress Cataloging-in-Publication Data

Safety in American Football/Earl F. Hoerner, editor.
    (STP; 1305)
    Papers presented at the Symposium on Safety in American Football,
hold in Phoenix, Arizona on 5–7 Dec. 1994.
    Includes bibliographical references and indexes.
    ISBN 0-8031-2400-7
    1. Football—United States—Safety measures—Congresses.
2. Football players—Wounds and injuries—United States—Prevention—
Congresses. I. Hoerner, Earl F. II. Symposium on Safety in
American Football (1994: Phoenix, Ariz.) III. Series: ASTM special
technical publication: 1305.
GV953.6.S35   1997
796.332—dc20   96-35836
                                                                      CIP

Photocopy Rights

Peer Review Policy

Each paper published in this volume was evaluated by two peer reviewers and at least
one of the Editors. The authors addressed all of the reviewers' comments to the
satisfaction of the technical editor(s) and the ASTM Committee on Publications.

The quality of the papers in this publication reflects not only the obvious efforts of the
authors and the technical editor(s), but also the work of these peer reviewers. The ASTM
Committee on Publications acknowledges with appreciation their dedication and
contribution to time and effort on behalf of ASTM.

Printed in Ann Arbor, MI
January 1997

Foreword

The Symposium on Safety in American Football was held in Phoenix, Arizona on 5–7 Dec. 1994. The sponsor of the event was ASTM Committee F-8 on Sports Equipment and Facilities. The symposium chairman was Earl F. Hoerner, and he also served as editor of this publication.

Contents

MANAGEMENT: SYSTEMS

Overview

Coaches, administrators, health and medical care providers are increasingly challenged to review and evaluate the risks associated with participating and playing in sports, including leisure time and recreational activities.

THE GAME
—What happens?
—Are there risks?
—Can risks be modified or limited?

To meet such challenges, these professionals must continue to examine, review and understand the scientific factors and infrastructure of the physical activity being studied. This information forms the underpinnings and circumstances of risk assessment, which includes within its discipline Epidemiology, Biomechanics, Ergonomics, Human Factors, Kinesiology, Tissue Tolerance, Environmental Studies, Materials, and Lifestyles. These factors represent but a few of the variables that must be considered in Risk Factor Assessment. The process of Risk Factor Assessment also encompasses the area of Biostatistics, utilizing new mechanistic and data distribution approaches to perform the role of assessment in managing risks, and communicating results to decision and policy makers as well as to the general public.

Focusing both on practical as well as integrated approaches, this Symposium Technical Proceeding is prepared to present some of the complex problems in the sport/athletic activity of American Football.

Earl F. Hoerner

Biomotions, Inc.,
Braintree, Massachusetts; symposium chairman and STP editor

Analyzing Risk

R. Glassman[1]

Barriers to Injury Prevention in Youth Football

REFERENCE: Glassman, R., "**Barriers to Injury Prevention in Youth Football,**" *Safety in American Football, ASTM STP 1305,* Earl F. Hoerner, Ed., American Society for Testing and Materials, 1996, pp. 3–8.

ABSTRACT: The National Youth Sports Safety Foundation (NYSSF), formerly the National Youth Sports Foundation for the Prevention of Athletic Injuries, a nonprofit, 501 (C) (3) educational research organization dedicated to reducing the number and severity of injuries youth sustain in sports activities, has been involved in injury prevention efforts in youth football since 1989. During that time the Foundation has traveled an eye-opening journey encountering many different barriers to injury prevention at all levels. These barriers include: (1) misinformation, (2) attitude, (3) dissemination of information, (4) lack of coaching education, and (5) surveillance.

Many injuries can be prevented through educational programs but there has to be a perceived need for these programs. There should be effective dissemination, follow-up, and evaluation systems in place.

KEYWORDS: injury prevention, dissemination, coaching education, surveillance, youth football

The NYSSF is a nonprofit, educational research organization working to promote the safety of children and adolescents participating in sports. Its mission is to reduce both the number and severity of injuries that youth sustain in sports activities. The Foundation serves as an educational resource and a clearinghouse of information on safe-sports participation for health professionals, program administrators, coaches, parents, and athletes. Its information comes from national medical organizations, sports organizations, journal articles, and leaders in the field.

The Foundation launched a national campaign in 1993, National Youth Sports Injury Prevention Month, (observed during the month of April) to promote safety in sports activities. The health event was supported by more than sixty national medical and sports organizations including the American Academy of Pediatrics, American College of Sports Medicine, United States Olympic Committee, Special Olympics, and The President's Council on Physical Fitness and Sports.

The Foundation publishes a quarterly newsletter, educational literature including fact sheets, resource sheets and guidelines, and provides the following services: national speakers bureau, conferences, coaching education clinics, bibliographic searches, and exhibit tables.

The NYSSF has been involved in injury prevention efforts in youth football since 1989. Since that time the Foundation has traveled an eye-opening journey encountering many different

[1]Associate executive director, National Youth Sports Safety Foundation, Ten Meredith Circle, Needham, MA 02192.

barriers to injury prevention at all levels. These barriers include: (1) misinformation, (2) attitude, (3) dissemination of information, (4) lack of coaching education, and (5) surveillance.

Misinformation as a Barrier

The Foundation has learned that there is a general misconception among program administrators and coaches of youth football regarding safety, injury prevention information, and resources. Repeatedly, the Foundation hears the following statements from youth football coaches:

- "Injuries are part of the game."
- "Injuries are not a problem."

From youth football program administrators we hear:

- "Our organization will be held to a higher standard if we are informed."

The administrator believes their coaches will be held to a higher standard if involved in litigation as a result of an injury sustained in their program if their group has the information. In fact, it is not unusual for youth football programs to shun presentations on safety for this reason. A safety program would include information on an emergency medical plan, an immediate first responder in case of injury, coaching education, and injury prevention.

In addition, many coaches and program administrators of youth football programs that are not affiliated with a national program do not know how to locate resources regarding safety and injury prevention.

Attitude as a Barrier

It has been our experience that although youth football organizations advocate the importance of safety, many areas relating to it still need to be addressed. Politics and tradition-bound resistance prevail. Many program administrators do not recognize the need for coaching education or injury prevention interventions and many worthwhile programs have not been utilized. The Foundation has frequently heard the following from them:

- "Don't tell them, you might scare them."
- "If coaches find out there are risks, they might not want to coach. We have enough trouble getting coaches."
- "If you tell parents there are risks, they won't let their children participate"; or "If you tell children there are risks, they won't want to play the game."

We also often hear, "Negative statements hurt sports and sports participation. It is not a responsible thing to do." For example, the head of a national youth football association would not use an injury prevention program on the risks of spearing because he felt it might scare the coaches. In addition, he felt that informing the players of the risks would scare them from the sport.

Many coaches we have spoken with do not feel there is a need to attend coaching clinics and sports medicine programs. They are very closed minded. Coaches know what they are going to do in their program and are not open to new material. They do not understand the need to keep current on the fast paced field of sports medicine. Coaches cling to the drills they learned from their coaches when they were players, and do not know that many of the exercises they are teaching are now considered to be contraindicated and place players at risk of injury.

Dissemination as a Barrier

Several years ago the Foundation received a memo from Dr. Joseph Torg from the University of Pennsylvania Sports Medicine Center [1]. Dr. Torg produced a video on preventing catastrophic neck and spine injuries which was funded by Riddell [2]. The video was distributed through the National Federation of State High School Associations [3] to its member state associations that were supposed to distribute them to local high schools. It was recommended that the video be mandatory viewing for all football coaches and students. However, working with the Adopt-A-School Program [4] (a program of the Urban Fitness Subcommittee of the Massachusetts Governor's Committee on Physical Fitness and Sports which has organized sports medicine clinics to provide pro bono treatment of injured interscholastic athletes in the Boston School System), the Foundation learned that not all high schools in the state of Massachusetts received a copy of the video or knew it even existed.

In addition, the Foundation learned that in one of the schools involved in the Adopt-A-School program, a high school football player sustained a catastrophic injury that left him paralyzed in Boston City Hospital. The young man was absent the day the coach showed Dr. Torg's tape on the dangers of spearing, and when the player returned to school, he did not have an opportunity to view it. The young man lowered his head when he went to tackle a player, speared him, and paid a very heavy price. The coach said in all his years of coaching he had never seen it happen, and didn't think it would ever happen to one of his players.

The Foundation wanted to learn more about the dissemination process of this excellent program and how it broke down. In the fall of 1994, the Foundation sent a survey to the executive directors of the 51 state high school athletic associations. Of the 51 associations surveyed, 37 responded. The following are the survey questions and responses.

(1) Did your state association receive a copy of the video, "Prevent paralysis: Don't hit with your head" to disseminate to your member schools?

- 14 replied no,
- 23 responded yes, and
- only three associations sent a copy of the video to each member school (DC, MO, WV).

Comments from the schools included:

- could not afford the cost,
- it was sent to schools upon request,
- each school had an opportunity to see the video,
- one association produced its own video,
- only 10% of schools play football.

(2) Whom was the video sent to?

- athletic director (MO, MT, and LA upon request),
- football coach (DC, LA upon request),
- principal (WV, LA upon request),
- football committee (NY, NM, NH), and
- other (two not specified).

(3) Was viewing the video made mandatory by the state high school association for the following groups?

- football coaches (six-DC, DE, MN, NC, NM, WV),

- players (two-DC, WV),
- officials (seven-AL, DE, LA, MN, NM, OR, WA).

(4) Was it up to each individual school as to whether or not they utilized the video?

- yes (15-AL, AK, DC, IA, LA, MA, MN, MS, MT, NC, OR, SC, SD, VA, WA), and
- no (two-DE, WV).

(5) If viewing the video was not mandatory in the past, are there any plans for it to be in the future for:

- football coaches (0),
- players (0), and
- officials (1-LA).

(6) Please rate your perceived value of this injury intervention program on the following scale: 1 = excellent, 5 = poor. Circle the number that best corresponds with the value of the program.

Scale Value	Number of Responses
• 1	(8)
• 2	(5)
• 3	(4)
• 4	(2)
• 5	(0)

(7) Have there been any catastrophic injuries sustained by students participating in high school football in member schools of your state association during the last two academic school years (catastrophic injury is defined as death or paralysis)?

- no (26), and
- yes (11-AL, CA, FL one paralysis one death, HI, IL, LA, MD, MA, NY, NC, WV one death).

The results of the survey clearly define the need for program administrators at the highest levels to advocate injury prevention as a high priority when they disseminate information on prevention programs.

Lack of Coaching Education

The United States is the only major country in the sporting world without a national coaching education program [5]. Less than 20% of the coaches in this country have had any formal training in coaching [5,6]. Fourteen states have no requirements at all to coach at the interscholastic level [7]. Of the states that do have requirements, there is no consistency among them. Some states require either a teaching certificate, certification in first aid/CPR, or certain college courses [8]. On the youth sports level, only New Jersey requires a course in liability.

Several coaching education programs have been developed and delivered nationally by independent groups. The most notable are: American Sport Education Program (ASEP) [9] which has been adopted by the National Federation of State High School Associations, Program on Athletic Coaching Education (PACE), [10] National Youth Sports Coaches Association program (NYSCA) [11]. The Foundation has been delivering the ASEP and NYSCA program for several years. However, both lack certain components that would optimize their effectiveness. These include:

(a) qualified individuals to teach the course,
(b) on-the-field instruction in technique and drills,
(c) internships, and
(d) evaluation components.

It has been our experience that the coaching education programs which are video-driven cram courses such as the above mentioned ones do not work effectively, and that coaches are not able to implement what they have learned.

While professional football has set a sterling example of taking every conceivable precaution in the event of injury to the extent of helivac for transportation [12], many youth sports football programs are being run without medical releases, emergency plans, and emergency response personnel. We have seen this countless number of times, especially in community youth sports programs that have no affiliation with national programs. Also, many youth sports and high school program administrators believe that medical coverage is only necessary for games; however, research has shown that in some sports more injuries occur in practices rather than in games [13–15]. In addition, it is our experience that coaches and program administrators have not recognized the need for continuing education.

Surveillance as a Barrier

"Despite the large number of sports-injury studies, most have been inconclusive due to inconsistent injury classification, lack of standardized reporting and recording techniques, and the failure to use appropriate statistical techniques to analyze the data" [16]. "Unfortunately, the standard classification scheme used in coding hospital discharge data does not identify most sports injuries" [17]. There is no mechanism in place to track all injuries effectively on the recreational level, high school level or youth sports level. Although we have had a surveillance system tracking catastrophic injuries in football, there are still many other vital areas which have not been addressed. One of the most critical in the Foundation's opinion is overuse injuries. Sports medicine clinics have reported an epidemic of overuse injuries; however, there is no system in place to track these. The government has not set this as a priority, however, because there is no statistical information or estimates on costs to the public.

Conclusion

At every conference, sports medicine night, and safety fair we have attended, many people come up to us and talk about their football injuries from their youth that have never left them and have restricted their participation in physical fitness activities. These injuries have contributed to health risk factors and affected the quality of their lives.

We have shown the barriers we have encountered in football injury prevention. How long will it take, and how many injuries must be sustained before sports injury prevention becomes a priority?

With the increase of children participating in organized sports at earlier and earlier ages, it is obvious that injuries have increased tremendously. All these injuries will become statistics. Every statistic has a name and a face and a story. Every statistic has a family who has agonized over the well-being of their child. And many statistics have families that have been burdened by surgery, rehabilitation, and financial expenses. Many of these injuries stay with players the rest of their lives, and force them to drop out of sports activities altogether.

The Foundation believes that sports participation may provide a very valuable experience for a child and that children are our greatest resource, but they deserve better. They deserve quality programs in which their safety and well-being are the number one priority. They deserve quality coaches who know how to teach the sport correctly, can recognize and prevent injuries, and give them a quality experience.

Myths abound regarding injuries and football. Although football is a contact sport and some injuries are inevitable, many still can be prevented through educational programs. But there has to be a perceived need for these programs from the top down. There must be effective dissemination, follow-up and evaluation systems in place.

References

[1]   Torg, J. S., University of Pennsylvania Sports Medicine Center, 235 South 33rd St., Philadelphia, PA 19104-9959.

[2]   Riddell, Inc., 3670 North Milwaukee Ave., Chicago, IL 60641.

[3]   National Federation of State High School Associations, 11724 N. W. Plaza Circle, Kansas City, MO 64195-0626.

[4]   Micheli, L. J., "Adopt-A-School Program," Urban Fitness Subcommittee, Massachusetts Governor's Committee on Physical Fitness and Sports. Dept. of Orthopaedics, The Children's Hospital, 300 Longwood Ave., Boston, MA 02115.

[5]   Dulberg, H., "Emotional Injuries in Youth Sports," *Sidelines*, Vol. 4, No. 2, 1995, pp. 1,2–4.

[6]   Kimiecik, J. C., "Who Needs Coaches' Education? US Coaches Do," *The Physician and Sports Medicine*, Vol. 16, No. 11, November 1988, pp. 124–134.

[7]   "Your Child Sports & Injuries, Do You Know the Risks?," National Youth Sports Foundation for the Prevention of Athletic Injuries, 1990.

[8]   Sisley, B. L. and Wiese, D. M., "Current Status: Requirements for Interscholastic Coaches," *JOPERD*, September 1987, pp. 75–85.

[9]   American Sport Education Program (ASEP), Box 5076, Champaign, IL 61820.

[10] Program on Athletic Coaching Education (PACE), Youth Sports Institute, I.M. Sports Circle Building, Room 213, Michigan State University, East Lansing, MI 489824.

[11] National Youth Sports Coaches Association (NYSCA), 2611 Old Okeechobee Road, West Palm Beach, FL 33409.

[12] Barnes, R. P., "Emergency Plan for Youth Sports," *Sidelines*, Vol. 3, No. 3, 1994, pp. 1–2.

[13] McLain, L. G. and Reynolds, S., "Sports Injuries in High School," *Pediatrics*, Vol. 84, No. 3, September 1989, pp. 446–450.

[14] "Youth Sports Injuries Fact Sheet," National Youth Sports Foundation for the Prevention of Athletic Injuries, Inc., 1993.

[15] Rowe, P. J. and Miller, L. K., "Treating High School Sports Injuries—Are Coaches/Trainers Competent?," *JOPERD*, January 1991, pp. 49–54.

[16] Whieldon, T. H. and Cerny, F. J., "Incidence and Severity of High School Athletic Injuries," *Athletic Training, JNATA*, 1990, pp. 344–350.

[17] Gallagher, S. S., "MA: A Case Example of How a Surveillance System Works," *Conference on Sports Injuries in Youth*, Bethesda, MD, April 1991, pp. 8–9.

Randall W. Dick[1]

A Comparison of Injuries That Occur During Collegiate Fall and Spring Football Using the NCAA Injury Surveillance System

REFERENCE: Dick, R. W., "A Comparison of Injuries That Occur During Collegiate Fall and Spring Football Using the NCAA Injury Surveillance System," *Safety in American Football, ASTM STP 1305,* Earl F. Hoerner, Ed., American Society for Testing and Materials, 1996, pp. 9–18.

ABSTRACT: The collegiate spring football season, which currently consists of five noncontact and ten contact practices, has been associated with a high incidence of injury. This study uses NCAA Injury Surveillance System (ISS) data to compare injury patterns in collegiate fall (FF) and spring (SF) football over the past four seasons. A reportable injury was defined as restricting the athlete's participating for at least one day. An athlete-exposure (A-E) was recorded for each individual participating in each practice or game. Results showed that the four-year practice injury rate for SF (9.0 injuries/1000 A-E) was more than double that of FF (4.0 injuries/1000 A-E). The top three types of injuries (knee, ankle, and shoulder) were identical in SF and FF with similar percentages of all reported injuries. Specific analysis of injury severity (time loss and required surgery), concussions, and new injuries also showed a higher rate in spring practice. There was little difference in the types of injuries that occurred in SF and FF: the SF injury incidence was just greater. Variables such as training, intensity, and recovery time may be factors in the increased SF injury rates. Reducing the number of contact practices in the spring may be one way of normalizing injury rates.

KEYWORDS: injury, spring football, fall football, noncontact

Division I and II National Collegiate Athletics Association (NCAA) football consists of two distinct seasons. The fall season, which begins with August practice and ends 3 to 4 months later with final regular season, postseason playoff or postseason bowl games, includes 10 to 14 games and multiple practices. The spring season consists exclusively of practices and scrimmages over a period of approximately a month. Proponents of the spring season cite the teaching of blocking and tackling fundamentals, evaluating nonscholarship players and players at new positions, and establishing starters for the fall season as justification for its existence. However, there may be a cost to these benefits in the form of injury. There is a perception that collegiate spring football is associated with a high incidence of injury, although there have been little published data in this regard [1].

The purpose of this study was to determine the injury rate in collegiate spring football and compare it with practice sessions in the fall season using the NCAA Injury Surveillance System (ISS). Only after definitive injury data are produced can the benefits and costs of spring football be effectively evaluated.

---

[1]Assistant director of Sports Sciences, National Collegiate Athletic Association. Overland Park, KS 66201.

Methods

Data Collection System

The NCAA Injury Surveillance System (ISS) was developed in 1982 to provide current and reliable data on injury trends in intercollegiate athletics [2]. Injury data are collected yearly from a representative sample of NCAA member institutions and the resulting data summaries are reviewed by the NCAA Committee on Competitive Safeguards and Medical Aspects of Sports. The committee's goal continues to be to reduce injury rates through suggested changes in rules, protective equipment, or coaching techniques based on data provided by the ISS.

During the 1982-1983 academic year, injury data were collected only on the sport of fall football. Since that time, the ISS has been expanded to include 15 additional sports. Spring football was added to the system in 1988.

Sampling

Participation in the NCAA Injury Surveillance System is voluntary and limited to the 893 member institutions (as of September, 1993). ISS participants are selected from the population of schools sponsoring a given sport. Selections are random within the constraints of having a minimum 10% representation of each NCAA division (I, II, and III) and region (East, South, Midwest, West). This sampling scheme assures a true cross-section of NCAA institutions that can be used to express injury rates representative of the total population of NCAA institutions sponsoring a particular sport.

It is important to emphasize that this system does not identify EVERY injury that occurs at NCAA institutions in a particular sport. Rather, it collects a sampling that is representative of a cross-section of NCAA institutions.

Data Reporting

Injury and exposure data are recorded by certified and student athletic trainers from participating institutions. Information is collected from the first official day of preseason practice to the final tournament contest.

Injuries

A reportable injury in the ISS is defined as one that:

1. Occurs as a result of participation in an organized intercollegiate practice or game;
2. Requires medical attention by a team athletic trainer or physician;
3. Results in restriction of the student-athlete's participation for one or more days beyond the day of injury.

A separate report is submitted for each injury by an athletic trainer. Each injury is described in detail including type of injury, body part injured, severity of injury, field type, field condition, and special equipment worn.

Exposures

To establish an injury rate, data are expressed as the number of injuries per unit of participation or risk.

An athlete exposure (A-E), the unit of risk in the ISS, is defined as one athlete participating in one practice or game where he or she is exposed to the possibility of athletic injury.

A one-page exposure form, submitted weekly, summarizes the number of practices and games, types of playing surfaces, and numbers of participants.

Injury Rate

An injury rate is simply a ratio of the number of injuries in a particular category to the number of athlete exposures in that category. In the ISS, this value is expressed as injuries per 1000 athlete exposures. For example, six reportable injuries during 563 athlete exposures results in an injury rate of (6/563) by 1000 or 10.7 injuries/1000 athlete exposures.

Fall Football Practice

NCAA legislation allows for a maximum of 29 practice opportunities before a school's first intercollegiate game. The first three practices must be noncontact; there are no further restrictions on type of practices. Once the regular season begins, a traditional Saturday game is *typically* followed by a light noncontact workout on Monday, more intensive contact work on the next three days, and a light noncontact day on Friday.

Spring Football Practice

NCAA legislation allows for a designated number of spring practice sessions within a defined period of time (22 to 29 days). In general, a certain percentage of these practices are designated as contact practices and often include scrimmages and one "spring game" while a lesser percentage are designated as noncontact.

The specific allowable spring practices since 1989 are shown in Fig. 1. Because a consistent schedule of 15 practices, ten of which may involve contact, has occurred since 1990, most of the data reported in this paper will involve the 1990 to 1993 period. However, it is important to note the differences in previous years, specifically the 12 "noncontact only" practices allowed in Division II in the 1989 to 1990 season.

Results

Figure 2 shows the practice injury rate in fall football since 1984 and in spring football since 1988. Since 1988, the spring injury rate has annually been more than twice that of fall practice.

SPRING FOOTBALL
1989 - 93

	Div. I	**Div. II**
1989 - 90	20 Practices	12 Practices
	15 Contact	0 Contact
1990 - 93	15 Practices	15 Practices
	10 Contact	10 Contact

FIG. 1—*Spring practice schedule by division 1989–1993.*

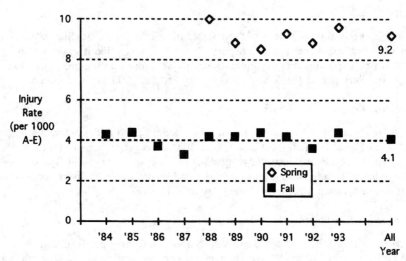

FIG. 2—*Spring and fall football practice injury rate 1984–1993.*

Figure 3 shows similar data in the 1990 to 1993 period. As noted above, this time frame will be analyzed in detail due to the consistent spring practice schedule.

Figure 4 shows the top three body parts injured in spring and fall football. The knee, ankle, and shoulder were the top body parts injured and were injured in similar percentages in the two activities.

Figure 5 shows the new injury rate in spring and fall football practice. Injuries were classified as new if no previous similar injury had been experienced in football or any other activity. The spring new injury rate over the four-year period was more than twice that of fall practice. Such injuries account for greater than 80% of all injuries in both activities.

Figure 6 shows the concussion injury rate in spring and fall football practice. The spring injury rate in this category is also more than twice that of fall practice.

Figures 7 and 8 show two measures of injury severity, both of which are approximately three times higher in spring practice. Figure 7 shows the rate of injury that caused at least seven days of restricted participation in fall and spring football practice. A limitation of this type of analysis is that injuries occurring at an end of a season or in the middle of a short season can only be estimated with regard to time loss.

Figure 8 shows the rate of injury that resulted in surgery. Limitations of this type of analysis are the changing nature and application of surgical methods and that some severe injuries, such as concussions, may not require surgery.

Figure 9 shows the Division II fall and spring practice injury rate since 1988. Note that the one year in which spring practice was restricted completely to noncontact (1989), the spring injury rate was almost identical to fall practice. The fall 1990 injury rate following noncontact spring practice was only slightly higher than the six-year average for the category.

Discussion

A four-year analysis of collegiate fall and spring football injuries using the NCAA Injury Surveillance System shows that spring practice has a consistent annual injury rate that is more

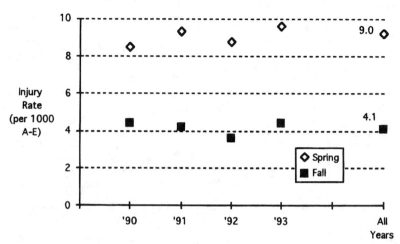

FIG. 3—*Spring and fall football practice injury rate 1990–1993.*

TOP 3 BODY PARTS INJURED
SPRING AND FALL FOOTBALL

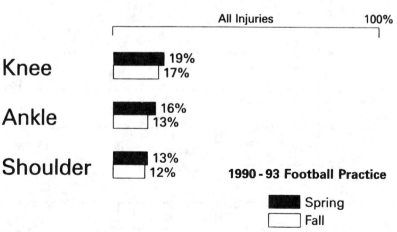

FIG. 4—*Spring and fall football top three body parts injured.*

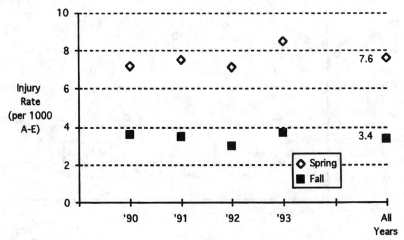

FIG. 5—*Spring and fall football new injury rate 1990–1993.*

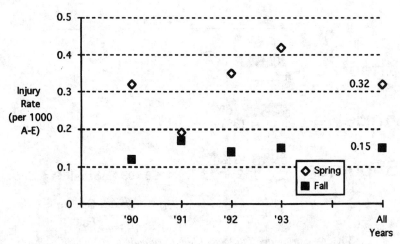

FIG. 6—*Spring and fall football concussion injury rate 1990–1993.*

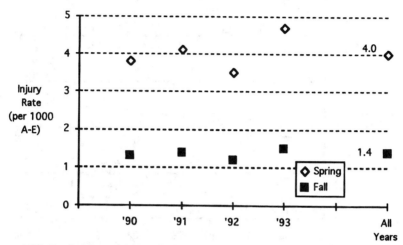

FIG. 7—*Spring and fall football 7+ days time loss injury rate 1990–1993.*

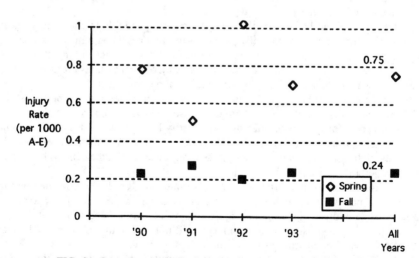

FIG. 8—*Spring and fall football surgery injury rate 1990–1993.*

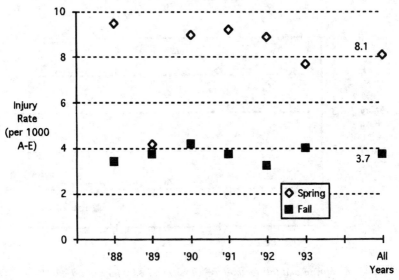

FIG. 9—*Division II spring and fall football practice injury rate 1988–1993.*

than twice that of fall practice. Assuming 75 individuals in each practice, the spring injury rate of 9.0 injuries per 1000 A-E equates to one injury every 1.5 practices. Using the same 75-player assumption, the fall injury rate of 4.0 equates to one injury every 3.3 practices. The types of injuries and body parts injured are similar in the two activities; the primary difference is the frequency of occurrence.

It has been pointed out by coaches that comparing spring and fall practice injury rates may be misleading. Since one is not formally preparing for a game, the argument goes, an athlete is much more likely to miss a spring practice or be held out of practice longer to be sure of complete recovery. In the fall, such a cushion is not available since one is preparing for games on a weekly basis. In this situation, playing "hurt" is more the norm.

Such an argument may be applicable to the injury severity category of time loss shown in Fig. 7. Time loss may be higher in the spring because one is more concerned about recovery for the fall season. However, other measures of severity like concussions (Fig. 6) and injuries requiring surgery (Fig. 8) are more absolute measures that include much less variability. Significantly higher spring practice rates in these categories support the conclusion that spring practice has certain increased risks of injury.

Another explanation for the differences in injury rates may be that injuries incurred in the fall season are not given enough time to heal prior to spring practice. The player is in a "weakened" state and the higher spring injury rate results from reoccurrence of an existing injury. Figure 5, however, shows that the injury rate difference in the spring and fall practices is evident even when comparing just new injuries.

Perhaps spring practice involves more contact, thereby causing a greater injury rate than fall practice. In the 1990 to 1993 period, spring practice involved 10 contact practices and five noncontact practices. Fall practices have fewer specific requirements regarding contact and noncontact. The first three fall preseason practices are required to be noncontact; typically a majority of the following 25 to 30 practices before the first game involve contact. Once the regular season starts, a typical scenario may involve two contact and three noncontact practices a week over a three-month period. Considering both the fall preseason and regular season frequency of contact practices, the ratio of contact to noncontact practices in both spring and fall practice is similar.

Coaches have also suggested that the type and intensity of contact occurring in spring and fall practices is different. A 1995 survey by the College Football Association (CFA) indicates that in the spring, teams average 3.4 game-type scrimmages in the allotted 10 contact practices [3]. Scrimmages have injury rates that resemble that of games; significantly higher than those of regular practices. The ratio of one game-type scrimmage every three contact spring practices is probably higher than what occurs in the fall. The greater relative frequency of this activity in the spring may contribute to the difference in practice injury rates. However, data from the Big-10 Conference, collected under a completely different system, indicate that the fall practice injury rate excluding scrimmages was more than double that of the spring practice excluding scrimmages [4]. Therefore, it appears that even when scrimmages are accounted for, contact practices in the spring elicit a greater number of injuries than those in the fall. Modification of the contact in spring practices may be a way to address this problem.

Figure 9 provides some insight into the injury rate difference between spring and fall practice. The 1989 spring practice in Division II consisted of 12 practices, all noncontact. The resulting injury rate was similar to that of the fall. In addition, the fall 1990 rate was not significantly higher than the six-year average for the category. These results lead to three important conclusions: (1) Contact has a significant effect on the injury rate in practice; one way to reduce injuries is to reduce contact, (2) reducing or eliminating contact in the spring does not appear to affect adversely the injury rate the following fall. There is some concern that altering spring practice would cause more intense fall practices to make up for what was missed in the spring, with a resulting increased injury rate and (3) noncontact practices reduce but do not eliminate injury. The spring 1989 injury rate in Fig. 9 was still similar to a fall injury rate consisting of both contact and noncontact practices. This may indicate a lack of compliance with the no contact rule, a lack of appropriate stretching or conditioning before the spring drills, or too little acclimatization to immediate intense physical activity.

Conclusion

Every sport has a baseline rate of injury that is associated with competing at a particular level. Such a level is normally established in the traditional playing season. Collegiate football has a unique situation that allows a defined out-of-season practice schedule. However, the benefit of this practice from a safety standpoint has been questioned because of a perceived injury risk that is substantially higher than what might be expected based on data associated with the traditional season.

An analysis of collegiate spring and fall football practice injury data indicate that spring football has a significantly higher injury rate, although both activities involve similar ratios of contact to noncontact practices. This finding is also apparent in specific categories of concussion, new injuries, time loss, and injuries requiring surgery. The types of injuries appear to be similar in the two activities, just occurring more frequently in the spring.

Variability in contact practice, such as scrimmages and intensity, may account for part of the seasonal injury differences. Analysis has shown that reducing contact is one way of affecting injury rates in football practice. Modification of contact may also be an option.

From this study, it can be concluded that spring football is associated with a significantly higher injury rate. Dialogue with football coaches is ongoing in factoring this "cost" against the benefits of teaching blocking and tackling fundamentals, evaluating walk-ons and players at new positions, and establishing starters for the fall season. To what extent safety recommendations can be applied before affecting skill development in a true contact sport remains to be seen.

References

[1] Clarke, K. S., "Spring Football Injury Report," *Athletic Administration,* Vol. 11, No. 3, 1977, pp. 16–21.

[2] NCAA Injury Surveillance System, c/o Randall W. Dick, Assistant Director of Sports Sciences, NCAA, 6201 College Boulevard, Overland Park, KS 66211.

[3] Personal correspondence, Neinas, C. M., Executive Director. College Football Association, 6688 Gunpark Drive, Suite 201, Boulder, CO 80301-3339.

[4] Personal correspondence, John W. Powell, University of Iowa Sports Medicine, Iowa City, Iowa, 52242.

Assessment

Leonard K. Lucenko[1]

Coaches Safety Orientation and Training Skills Program

REFERENCE: Lucenko L. K., **"Coaches Safety Orientation and Training Skills Program,"** *Safety in American Football, ASTM STP 1305,* Earl F. Hoerner, Ed., American Society for Testing and Materials, 1996, pp. 21–31.

ABSTRACT: Coaching is one of the crucial elements in the conduct of safe play in football at every level. The coach can have the greatest impact on safety and must be educated to make safety a priority in team management.

There is a trend in the professional education of coaches to reduce the professional preparation course work and to hire coaches with minimal education and training. On the recreational level, coaching credentials are minimal at best.

This paper explores the problems encountered in the coaching environment relating to football safety and the steps being taken to improve coaching education. The model used, herein, is the New Jersey State Legislation regarding the requirement for a program of "Safety and Skills Orientation" for volunteer coaches. It further proposes and recommends additional education and training for football coaches on all levels of play.

KEYWORDS: safety, football, liability, injuries, prevention, coaching, safety education

High school football accounted for the greatest number of direct catastrophic injuries for the fall sports, but high school football was also associated with the greatest number of participants. There are approximately 1 500 000 high school and junior high school football players participating each year.

The poignant and sobering video produced by Dr. Joseph Torg clearly states that the catastrophic injuries sustained by many football players are definitely preventable [1]. This must also be stated regarding most other injuries that occur during practice or game competition on the football field. Coaches need to be convinced of this fact so that an injury-preventing approach becomes part of their coaching philosophy and methodology. Additionally, they must instill injury prevention into every action and reaction of their players. Unfortunately, not all coaches are convinced that this must be part of their program.

The litigation explosion has brought to light many problems associated with coaching, and has resulted in demands by various public groups to educate coaches regarding sport safety and appropriate coaching methods. These lawsuits have defined the expectations of individuals in coaching roles and have put all coaches on notice that they are responsible to establish and conduct a safe athletic experience for their players.

It is an expectation of parents that when their child is enrolled in an athletic program, the coach is qualified and will have the welfare of the child as a primary responsibility. When this obligation or duty is violated by the coach, resulting in an injury to the child, lawsuits are inevitable. The best posture for coaches in preventing injuries and avoiding litigation is

[1] Professor, Montclair State University, Department of Health, Physical Education and Recreation, Upper Montclair, NJ 07043.

to understand their responsibilities as per "in loco parentis" and their roles as supervisors and teachers [2].

The New Jersey State Legislature has seen this as an important part of coaching education and has passed legislation to provide liability immunity to youth and volunteer football coaches if they undergo a safety and orientation training program. The legislation states:

> In order to be covered by the provisions for civil immunity as prescribed by New Jersey P.L. 1988, Chapter 87 (c.2A: 62A–6.2) the volunteer athletic coach, manager, or official must participate in a safety orientation and training skills program which meets the following minimally acceptable standards. These standards apply for all New Jersey volunteer athletic coaches, for all age groups, and for all populations of athletes served. [3]

Although the law falls in the category of enabling legislation, recreation departments and some school districts have strengthened its implementation. Those public entities that provide facilities for games and practices have required the safety and orientation training to issue a permit for the use of the facilities. No outside group that applies for a facility use permit is issued one without the coaches' training. All public recreation departments that sponsor "in-house" programs require the coaches to be trained.

The law does not cover any coaches involved in a public or private school athletic program, whether or not they are volunteers. School coaches are not covered. It is unfortunate that the law does not require coaches who do not have a college degree to undergo a skill and orientation training. New Jersey has a system that has developed the "60-credit wonder" *as a coach*. It provides that anyone who has completed any college courses totaling 60 credits can be hired as an assistant or head coach at a high school. No education in coaching principles, sports psychology, growth and development, fitness conditioning, or methods of teaching sports skills is required.

This system shows just as much of a need to educate high school coaches as to educate youth coaches.

The full text of the legislation is included in the Appendix.

Coaching Education for Safety

Institutions such as Montclair State University have felt encouraged to establish and conduct these programs.

The Montclair State University Coaching Academy is dedicated to the training of coaches in *Safety Orientation and Training Skills Programs*. The programs meet the requirements of P.L. 1988 c. 87 as enacted by the New Jersey Legislature to provide immunity from liability for damages in civil actions arising out of sports activities.

The Academy's safety orientation and skills training program meets the standards established by the Governor's Council on Physical Fitness and Sports, thereby providing the youth and recreational coach protection from liability.

The content of the New Jersey State Legislation, P.L. 1988, Chapter 87(c.2A:62A-6.2), that has been adapted by the Montclair State University Coaching Academy is as follows.

Medical, Legal, and First Aid Aspects of Coaching

Every volunteer coach/manager education program shall include basic knowledge and skills in the recognition and prevention of athletic injuries and knowledge of first aid. To ensure the standards are achieved, the following topics shall be included:

(1) legal and ethical responsibilities of the coach,

(2)   recognition of common sports injuries specific to the populations served by the sports programs,

(3)   safety plans and procedures for injury prevention, and

(4)   safety issues specific to the populations serviced.

Legal and Ethical Responsibilities of Football Coaches

The term, *coach,* comprises many responsibilities that have evolved from the general to the specific. Early responsibilities of the coach were limited to organization and training of the team members. Today the responsibilities have evolved into more formalized duties. They have been identified and prescribed, written and evaluated to include risk management and avoidance of unreasonable risk of injury to players. Performance in coaching has to be according to a *standard* and in avoidance of negligent action. This is accomplished by the recognition of risks and taking avoidance strategies to prevent injuries at all times while the players are under a coach's supervision.

The collision nature of football requires coaches to have a heightened sensitivity for safe preparation of the players, and for the execution of safe skills and tactics. Catastrophic injuries must be prevented at all costs. According to Dr. Torg, most can be prevented [4]. Coaches cannot take a cavalier attitude, stating that because football is a volunteer program and a young person elects to play the game, that young person assumes all responsibility for his or her safety.

Montclair State University Coaching Academy teaches that legal duties for coaches have been established by sports safety experts as well as by courts in litigation and include the following:

Proper Supervision—The coach is responsible for providing general as well as specific supervision throughout the coaching session or when the coach assumes responsibility for the players. General supervision includes overall direction of the work of the team. Specific supervision dictates the coach be with one or several players in close proximity and directly supervising the specific skill and technique in which they are engaged.

Among the important roles of the coach in respect to supervision are the following:

(a)   presence throughout the activity session and until players have departed;

(b)   supervisory plan developed, published, and implemented;

(c)   equipment and facility inspection to detect hazards and to anticipate problems; and

(d)   praise and appropriate communication.

Instruction—This responsibility requires the coach to have up-to-date knowledge of the sport. It is important to attend workshops, symposia, and clinics regularly to maintain and improve knowledge and skills. Coaching certification and safety orientation programs are available and should be attended. These are available from leagues, governing bodies, university programs, and service organizations.

The instruction, coaching, or teaching process of skills, techniques, and tactics includes knowing the proper techniques, proper progression, and providing feedback. A recommended progression for teaching fundamental game-related or game-condition phases includes the following:

(a)   organization of the team,

(b)   introduction of topic and communication of importance in game and safety aspects,

(c)   correct demonstration of skill to be learned: *A picture is worth a thousand words,*

(d) repeat demonstration—solidify the proper aspects,
(e) short and clear explanation,
(f) provide sufficient time for practice,
(g) feedback, solidification, modification,
(h) teachable moment—use the moment to make an important point, and
(i) review.

Position specific skill training and fitness conditioning—There are programs in New Jersey players play on offense and defense. Dr. Torg has identified positions that are most *at risk*. It is, therefore, the responsibility of the coach to make certain that adequate skill, tactical training, and fitness conditioning is provided to each player in each position he will play. A quarterback who spends 70% of his practices on offense and then practices 30% as a linebacker will be at risk to injury when playing on defense. Adequate instruction and practice time under supervision is imperative in this type of situation. Adequate practice promotes player game readiness and develops confidence. Lack of practice develops a lack of confidence and promotes indecision as well as improper and dangerous skill execution.

Dr. Torg, through his research, has reinforced that blocking and tackling are the two most hazardous skills in football that lead to the most serious injuries and quadriplegia. The National Collegiate Athletic Association (NCAA) in its *Sports Medicine Handbook* [5], also addresses the importance of appropriate football blocking and tackling in its policy.

"POLICY NO. 16: FOOTBALL BLOCKING AND TACKLING

Serious head and neck injuries leading to death, permanent brain damage or quadriplegia (extensive paralysis from injury to the spinal cord at the neck level) occur each year in football. The number is relatively small (less than one fatality for every 100,000 players and an estimated two to three nonfatal severe brain and spinal cord injuries for every 100,000 players), but constant. The injuries cannot be prevented completely due to the tremendous forces occasionally encountered in football collisions, but they can be minimized by helmet manufacturers, coaches, players, and officials complying with the accepted safety standards and the playing rules.

The rules against butting, ramming, and spearing with the helmet are for the protection of the helmeted player as well as his opponent. The player who does not comply with these rules is a candidate for a fatality or a catastrophic injury.

The American Football Coaches Association, emphasizing that the helmet is for the protection of the wearer and should not be used as a weapon, addresses the ramming, butting, and spearing situation in its Code of Ethics as follows [6]:

a. The helmet shall not be used as the brunt of the contact in the teaching of blocking or tackling.
b. Self-propelled mechanical apparatuses shall not be used in the teaching of blocking and tackling.
c. Greater emphasis by players, coaches and officials should be placed on eliminating spearing.

Proper training in tackling and blocking techniques constitutes an important means of minimizing the possibility of head injury and must be adequately addressed during each practice.

Rule changes—Administrators, coaches, and sports-governing organizations have a responsibility to evaluate constantly the circumstances of injuries and to implement rule changes to promote safety in the sport. A clear example of positive results of rule changes came about when the National Federation of State High School Associations and the NCAA changed football rules to *prevent spearing* and to *get the head out of football*. The result has been a drastic reduction of catastrophic injuries in the form of fatalities or quadriplegia. In 1992, there were four injuries that resulted in permanent paralysis spine injuries compared to 25 to 30 cases of these types of injuries in the early 1970s.

Rule changes must be implemented into the daily team management of each football coach. Coaches must teach skills and techniques according to the rules.

Head and neck injuries—The AFCA, the NCAA, and the Federation of State High School Associations (FSHSA) [7], in their annual survey of football injury research, have made recommendations for coaches for the prevention of injuries. First and foremost in the recommendations is the *elimination of the head as a primary and initial contact area for blocking and tackling.* The following are their suggestions for reducing head and neck injuries:

1. Athletes must be given proper conditioning exercises which will strengthen their necks so that participants will be able to hold their heads firmly erect when making contact.
2. Coaches should drill the athletes in the proper execution of the fundamental football skills, particularly blocking and tackling. Contact should always be made with the head up and never with the top of the head/helmet. Initial contact should never be made with the head/helmet.
3. Coaches and officials should discourage the players from using their heads as battering rams when blocking and tackling. The rules prohibiting spearing should be enforced in practice and in games. The players should be taught to respect the helmet as a protective device and that the helmet should not be used as a weapon.
4. All coaches, physicians, and trainers should take special care to see that the player's equipment is properly fitted, particularly the helmet.
5. When a player has experienced or shown signs of head trauma (loss of consciousness, visual disturbances, headache, inability to walk correctly, obvious disorientation, memory loss), he should receive immediate medical attention and should not be allowed to return to practice or game without permission from the proper medical authorities [8].

Warnings and Cautions—Team members and their parents need to be warned constantly of the known or inherent risks of the sport. This must be an ongoing process, not an infrequent occurrence. Daily instructions in safety is a requirement. The failure to warn the players of the dangers of using an improper technique can lead to injuries and litigation problems.

A Safe Coaching Environment—This duty includes the use of safe equipment or safe facilities. All necessary and required protective equipment must be worn by the players. The coach must make certain that the equipment itself is safe and fits properly. An inspection system should be implemented to check the equipment on a regular basis during its life. A daily check of the equipment is more appropriate than only a pre-season or post-season inspection. Any defect should be repaired, or the equipment should be replaced. Coaches should warn players not to misuse or abuse the equipment and use it only for the purpose intended.

Protective equipment—Coaches should follow the principles established by the governing bodies. These principles should be in effect during practices as well as competitive games and should be part of a continuous process of safety in the team environment. The *NCAA Sports Medicine Handbook* outlines the coach's responsibility regarding protective equipment.

The head coach or his designated representative shall certify to the umpire before the game that all players are equipped in compliance with NCAA football rules and:

(a)   have been informed what equipment is mandatory by rule and what constitutes illegal equipment,
(b)   have been provided the equipment mandated by rule,
(c)   have been instructed to wear and how to wear mandatory equipment during the game, and

(d) have been instructed to notify the coaching staff when equipment becomes illegal through play during the game.

The following list includes rules concerning protective and mandatory equipment:

(a) four-point chin strap with all snaps secured,
(b) soft knee pads at least one-half inch thick worn over the knees,
(c) an intra-oval mouthpiece that covers all upper jaw teeth,
(d) hip pads must have a tailbone protector,
(e) helmet that is NOCSAE approved,
(f) shoulder pads, thigh guards,
(g) all casts and splints are permissible only to protect an injury and must be properly padded on all sides, and
(h) therapeutic or preventive knee braces are permitted if covered from direct external exposure.

The National Athletic Trainees Association as well as other organizations have developed helmet fitting protocols which must be followed. All safety and protective equipment must be properly fitted. Helmets should have the National Operating Committee for Safety in Athletic Equipment (NOCSAE) stamp.

New protective and safety equipment that has been developed should be considered for adoption. Research and evaluation should be reviewed.

Facilities—Facilities should be inspected daily to detect any defects. Any defects detected should be corrected before use. The following is a recommended policy for facility risk management:

(1) inspect for hazards,
(2) detect the hazards,
(3) eliminate the hazards when possible,
(4) secure the hazards if they cannot be eliminated, and
(5) produce no additional hazards.

Proper football field maintenance is one of the critical areas in the prevention of football injuries during practices and games. The intense use of the football field, especially during daily practice sessions, requires a comprehensive seasonal, weekly, and daily maintenance program for safe use. The coach should be part of this system in providing information to the maintenance staff following a postpractice inspection of the fields. Proper liaison and mainte- nance steps will reduce potential injuries to players.

Health and Injury Care—A preparticipation exam is necessary because it provides detailed information regarding the players' current health status, physical fitness, and a history of illness, injury, or surgery [9]. If health problems are discovered during the exam, the player will be able to secure medical care to rehabilitate the cause. If it is not possible to treat the condition, and it is hazardous, the player will be so advised and prevented from participating.

Emergency first aid care for an injured athlete will generally fall to the coach, unless an athletic trainer is present. In most youth coaching sessions, there are no trainers present. There should be a first-aid kit at every practice and game [10]. The coach should be trained in first aid and CPR and should establish an emergency medical plan to provide reasonable medical assistance to injured participants as quickly as possible.

The emergency medical plan—The plan should be developed specifically for the team, league, and practice or game facility and include communication requirements with the local physicians and hospital.

The National Youth Sports Foundation has developed an Emergency Medical Plan that contains the following critical information necessary for appropriate immediate medical assistance [*11*]:

DESIGNATED PERSONNEL
1. Person designated to stay with injured athlete:
2. Person designated to phone for medical assistance:
3. Person designated to meet emergency medical assistance at gate and accompany them to injured athlete (This person should have all necessary keys to gates and doors in their possession):
4. Person designated to immediately call parents and inform them of circumstances:
5. Person designated to accompany injured athlete to the hospital:
6. Person responsible for documenting all information relating to injury and emergency response:

EMERGENCY INFORMATION
1. Location of closest phone:
2. Keys to access phone are located at:
3. Change for pay phone is kept in:
4. Address of the athletic facility is:
5. Entry location for the closest emergency vehicle is:
6. To access the athletic facility, emergency medical personnel must pass through _____ gates and _____ doors. Keys to unlock these areas are available from:
7. Phone number of emergency facility if 911 is not available:
8. The closest emergency care facility is _____ which is located at _____ and is _____ miles from the athletic facility. Average travel time is: _____.
9. The closest Trauma I facility is _____ which is located at _____ and is _____ miles from the athletic facility. Average travel time is: _____.

EMERGENCY CALL INSTRUCTIONS

When you call an emergency medical service (911), you should:

• Identify yourself and your exact location.
• Explain what happened and the type of injury (head, neck).
• Give address of athletic facility and exact instructions on how the ambulance is to reach the injured athlete. Include street address, gate information, building location, and entry information.
• Stay on the line until the operator disconnects the call.
• Return to the injury scene.

ADDITIONAL PHONE NUMBERS
Team Physician:
Ambulance Service:
Fire Department:
Police Department:
School Nurse:
Athletic Director:
Principal:

The Emergency Medical Plan must be issued to all coaches and parents of the players. There should be review and practice or rehearsal of the plan as if an injury actually occurred.

Postrehabilitation and Return to Competition—Parental and medical clearance is necessary before the player is permitted to participate again. The coach should not coerce nor intimidate the player to return to active participation before clearance has been given.

Examples of Coaching Problems in Football—The following are some examples that occurred in high school football and which can occur in youth football, which need to be addressed and incorporated into ongoing coaching education, in-service training, and/or CEU programs for football safety.

Preseason Scrimmage—A recent controversy at a New Jersey high school clearly shows that there are coaches who are not committed to a *safety* environment. The football coach scheduled a preseason scrimmage before meeting the **minimum** requirements for fitness and conditioning preparation as required by the New Jersey State Interscholastic Athletic Association. This disregard of an important safety protection rule for the high school football player indicates a need for a mechanism to educate the coach regarding the legal and ethical ramifications of his decision.

Captains' Practices—Recent revelations of abuses of new and inexperienced players have brought forth a need for the football coach to make certain that fitness and conditioning are the main considerations in the sessions. Some captains' sessions have included hazing and vicious, unexpected contact that resulted in injuries.

Although a coach is usually not present during the captains' practices, the coach has given the sessions his imprimatur and is responsible for providing information as a structure for the sessions, including safety.

Mismatching and Coaching Ethics—A courageous football coach at a high school requested that the school drop a long-time traditional rival because of inequalities in the players at the schools that included many components of athleticism as well as the numbers of players who were on the team. Additionally, the squad size was small and such that there was no opportunity for players to rest because most had to go both ways. Injuries were not given adequate time to heal before the next game and were due to the fatigue factor. The fatigue factor was explained by Dr. Fred Mueller in his comment, appropo to the above situation. "By the fourth quarter a team that has been playing the same personnel against a team that has been freely substituting will show signs of fatigue which could result in dropping the head when making a tackle" [*12*].

Other coaches have dealt with similar problems. Coaches of three high schools in New York protested promotion to a higher division of competition because they were concerned about the balance in the competition. One coach was quoted as saying, "I don't have a defeatist attitude . . . every school should play within its means. Balanced competition creates safer games . . ."

Conclusion

Football coaches occupy an important place in the lives of athletes. Many coaches have little formal coaching education. This missing component, however, does not absolve the coach if his actions result in injuries to his players. A program such as is in existence at the Montclair State University Coaching Academy provides education and training regarding all aspects of coaching responsibilities with special emphasis on coaching safety.

Appendix

The following is excerpted from the complete text of New Jersey State Legislation for Coaches Safety Orientation and Training Skills Program. P.L. 1988, c 87 (NJSA 2A:62A-6 et seq).

Chapter 52

Governor's Council on Physical Fitness and Sports

Subchapter 1. Minimum Standards for Volunteer Coaches' Safety Orientation and Training Skills Programs.

5.52. Introduction

(a) The minimum standards set forth in this subchapter identify the major topics which must be addressed in volunteer coaching/managing/officiating programs for safety orientation and training skills program required for civil immunity according to N.J.S.A. 2A: 62A-6 et seq. The topics must be presented within the context of an educational program that addresses the perspective of the specific population(s) or athletes served (for example, young, senior, disabled, novice and skilled athletes).

(b) In order to be covered by the provisions for civil immunity as prescribed by New Jersey P.L. 1988, c. 87 (N.J.S.A. 2A: 62A-6 et seq), the volunteer athletic coach, manager, or official must attend a safety orientation and skills training program of at least a three-hour duration which meets the minimum standards set forth in the subchapter. The programs may be provided by local recreation departments, non-profit organizations, and national/ state sports training organizations. The standards apply to all volunteer athletic programs in New Jersey regardless of populations served.

(c) Any organization providing a safety orientation and skills training program pursuant to these rules shall issue a certificate of participation to each participant who successfully completes the program.

5:52-1.2 Medical, legal and first-aid aspects of coaching.

(a) Every volunteer coach/manager educational program shall include basic knowledge and skills in the recognition and prevention of athletic injuries and knowledge of first aid. To ensure the standards are achieved the following topics shall be included:

1. Legal and ethical responsibilities of the coach;
2. Recognizing common sports injuries specific to the populations served by the sports program;
3. Safety plans and procedures for injury prevention;
4. Safety issues specific to the population serviced;
5. Plans and procedures for emergencies; and
6. Care and treatment of injuries generally associated with athletic activities.

5:52-1.3 Training and conditioning of athletes

(a) Every volunteer athletic coach/manager educational program shall include instruction in procedures for training and physical conditioning for participation in athletic activities appropriate for the population served. To ensure the standards are achieved, the following topics shall be included:
1. General principles of fitness and conditioning; and
2. Safety issues specific to environmental conditions in sport (for example, age, skill level, overtraining and staleness).

5:52-1.4 Psychological aspects of coaching

(a) Every volunteer athletic coach/manager educational program shall stress the importance of fostering positive social and emotional environments for all sports participants. To ensure the standards are achieved, the following topics shall be included:

1. Philosophy of coaching;
2. Psychological understanding of the individual athlete; and
3. Sportsmanship.

5:52-1.5 General coaching concepts

(a) Every volunteer athletic coach/manager educational program shall include general concepts of teaching and coaching athletic activities. To ensure the standards are achieved, the following topics shall be included:

1. Goals and objectives appropriate for the population served;
2. Teaching and coaching methods;
3. Planning and managing practices and competitions;
4. Coaching fundamental sports skills; and
5. The importance of playing rules.

5:52-1.6 General officiating concepts

(a) Every volunteer athletic official's educational program shall be designed to prepare the official to conduct a safely officiated, competitive experience based upon the rules of the game and the maturity level and proficiency of the athletes involved. To ensure the standards are achieved, the following topics shall be included:

1. Legal and ethical responsibilities of the official;
2. Safety issues under the control of the official;
3. Mechanics of officiating; and
4. Plans and procedures for medical emergencies.

References

[1] Torg, J., "Prevent Paralysis," Video, Riddell Inc., Chicago, IL., 1989.
[2] Lucenko, L. K., "Safety/Liability in Physical Education and Sport," *Communique,* Panzer Alumni, Montclair State University, Upper Montclair, NJ, 1994.
[3] State of New Jersey, "Volunteer Coaches Safety Orientation and Training Skills Program," PL 1988 c. 87, Trenton, NJ, 1988.
[4] Torg, J. S., Truex, R., Jr., Quedenfeld, T. C., et al. "The National Football Head and Neck Injury Registry Report and Conclusions 1978." *JAMA,* Vol. 6, 241, 1979, pp. 1477–1479.
[5] *Sports Medicine Handbook,* National Collegiate Athletic Association, Mission, KS, 1992.

[6] Mueller, F. "Tackle Football," in *Administration and Supervision for Safety and Sports,* American Alliance for Health, Physical Education, and Recreation, Washington, DC, 1977.

[7] Mueller, F. O. and Canty, R. C., *Annual Survey of Catastrophic Football Injuries, 1977–1992,* National Center for Catastrophic Injuries, Chapel Hill, NC, 1993.

[8] Mueller, F. O. and Schindler, R. D., *Annual Survey of Football Injury Research: 1931–1992,* National Center for Catastrophic Injuries, Chapel Hill, NC, 1993.

[9] Stepp, S. and Shankman, G., "Pre-Season Physicals Help Prevent Injuries," *Sport Care and Fitness,* 1989.

[10] *Sports Medicine: Health Care for Young Athletes,* American Academy of Pediatrics, Chicago, IL, 1991.

[11] *"Emergency Plan,"* National Youth Sports Foundation for the Prevention of Injury, Needham, MA, 1992.

[12] *Eleventh Annual Report,* National Center for Catastrophic Sports Injury Research, Chapel Hill, NC, 1993.

Barry Goldberg[1]

Injury in Youth Football

REFERENCE: Goldberg, B., "**Injury in Youth Football**," *Safety in American Football, ASTM STP 1305,* Earl F. Hoerner, Ed., American Society for Testing and Materials, 1996, pp. 32–34.

ABSTRACT: The participation of children and young adolescents in the sport of football has been an area of concern for parents and physicians. This concern has arisen from the well-documented risk of catastrophic and chronic disabling injuries that occur in high school, college, and professional competition. The smaller size and slower speed of young football players suggest that the reduced force of impact might create a different injury experience than that found at higher levels of competition. This paper will examine the injury experience of children participating in three divisions determined by weight and age.

KEYWORDS: football, youth, injuries, incidents, biostatistics, prevention, epidemiology

The participation of children and young adolescents in the sport of football has been an area of concern for parents and physicians. This concern has arisen from the well-documented risk of catastrophic and chronic disabling injuries that occur in high school, college, and professional competition [1–6]. The presence of an open epiphysis on the long bones in children represents another area of concern. The smaller size and slower speed of young football players suggest that the reduced force of impact might create a different injury experience than that found at higher levels of competition. Studies to assess this hypothesis were very limited [7,8] so in 1981, we began to study [9,10] the injury experience in Pop Warner Football, a league for players divided into divisions from age 8 to 15 years and from 22.5 to 67.5 kg. A pilot study was performed in 1981 and a more definitive study in 1983.

A pilot study examined the injury experience of 436 children participating in three divisions determined by weight and age. Sixty-seven injuries occurred, representing 15.4% of the population. Minor injuries (requiring less than seven days of restriction) accounted for 9.7% of the injuries, whereas 5.7% were significant (requiring more than seven days of restriction). Within the significant injury group, 3.2% of the total population sustained moderate injuries (7 to 21 days of restriction) and 2.5% sustained major injuries (>21 days of restriction). No severe injuries (resulting in permanent disability) occurred. Players of heavier weight sustained a significantly higher incidence and severity of injury. Members of the Pee Wee Division (ages 9 to 12, weight 29.3 to 45 kg) had an injury rate of 8.4%, of the Jr. Midget Division (age 10 to 13, weight 36 to 51.8 kg) 12.7%, and of the Midget Division (ages 11 to 14, weight 40.5 to 60.8 kg) 23.9%.

Sprains (34.3%) were the most prevalent injury followed by contusion (22.4%) and fractures (14.9%). The knee was the site most frequently injured (22.4%) followed by the hand/wrist (20.9%). The more serious injuries occurred most frequently to the hand/wrist and knee. Strains were rarely significant, and the tibia/fibula was the site most frequently fractured. Two epiphyseal fractures occurred and three players required hospitalization, two for concussions

[1]Director, Sport Medicine, Yale University Health Service, 17 Hillhouse Ave., North, New Haven, CT 06520.

and one for a reduction of an epiphyseal fracture. No internal knee derangement occurred. The positions most frequently and seriously injured included running back followed by defensive line and offensive line. Game (34) and practice (34) injuries were equal and contact was responsible for 62 of the 67 injuries. Coaches evaluated 28 of the 67 injuries, and few players (8) returned later to participation with physician's consent.

Subsequent to the pilot study, a larger study of 5,128 youth football players was undertaken during the 1983 season and children in 5 divisions ranging in age from 8 to 15 years and in weight from 22.5 to 67.5 kg were evaluated. Only significant injuries were recorded, and 257 injuries or 5% of the population sustained this magnitude of injury. Of the injured group, 61.1% incurred moderate injuries, and 38.9%, major injuries. Eight of the injuries were potentially severe, but at the conclusion of the study, only a cartilaginous injury of the knee had a significant risk of long-term disability. Hospitalization was required for 17 injuries, five of which required surgery including reduction of an epiphyseal fracture, an ankle, elbow, radius fracture, and a ruptured spleen.

The hand/wrist was most frequently injured (27.6%) followed by the knee (18.7%) and the shoulder/humerus (11.3%). The upper extremity was the site of most major injuries. Fracture (35%), sprains (24.5%), and contusions (16.7%) were most frequently diagnosed, and epiphyseal fractures accounted for 5% of the injuries. Only one injury to the knee resulted in an internal derangement. Weight and playing time were significantly related to injury although no significant correlation was found with age, experience, or a prior injury. Most injuries occurred in games (61.5%), and the majority were caused by direct contact (96%), most often player-to-player contact while tackling or running with the ball. The position of the players most often injured included running back (30.4%), defensive line (22.2%), and offensive line (12.8%). A significantly disproportionate number of major injuries occurred on kick-off and punt returns. Coaches evaluated 33.1% of the injuries whereas paraprofessionals evaluated 62.6%. Fifty-five players who returned immediately to participation neither reported their injury to any adult nor notified the coach that they were returning to the game.

There have not been any recent studies of youth football. The studies described provided the following information and observations:

(1) The 5% rate of significant injury is well below what was found at higher levels of competition.

(2) The upper body rather than the lower body appears to be at greatest risk of injury.

(3) Significant strains and sprains are much less common than at higher levels of competition, and internal derangements of the knee are rare.

(4) Catastrophic injuries did not occur and according to Jon Butler, of Pop Warner Football, no catastrophic football related injuries have occurred since his appointment as Executive Director in 1991, or to his knowledge after the 1983 study. No new significant rule changes have been implemented.

(5) Epiphyseal fractures account for 3 to 5% of all injuries, and all such injuries incurred were expected to heal with no residual damage.

(6) Running backs and offensive linemen were most often injured as compared to receivers and cornerbacks at older levels of competition.

(7) The incidence of injury in games was greater than in practice despite a shorter exposure time. Players who participated in most of a game sustained a greater number of injuries than substitutes.

(8) Current age and weight classifications for divisional play appear to be appropriate, as younger and lighter players did not experience an increased risk of injury.

(9) Coaches are frequently called on to evaluate injuries and determine if a child can return to competition.

(10)   Children will frequently not report injuries to coaches and will return to competition without permission.

The studies suggested changes that could potentially reduce the rate of injury.

(1)   With 8.2% of injuries occurring during contact drills, a reduction in the amount of contact practice should be considered.
(2)   As a disproportionate number of major injuries occurred on kick-off and punt returns, this aspect of the game could be eliminated.
(3)   Late hits and piling-on were responsible for 8.6% of the injuries, suggesting that officials become more aggressive in controlling the game.
(4)   An adult should be assigned to observe, evaluate, and control injured players so that they cannot return to competition without appropriate evaluation.
(5)   Modifications and improvement in equipment should continue, particularly of helmets, which, upon contact, caused 18.4% of the injuries.
(6)   Coaches are required to evaluate a large number of injuries without professional support and therefore should be educated and certified to assume this important role.
(7)   Pop Warner should consider implementing these findings which, to date, have been done on a local league level. The information from these studies were distributed by Pop Warner for local leagues.

Youth football represents an activity for children that has a significantly lower risk of injury than higher level of competition. The severity of the injuries sustained are also less. Therefore, the injury experience of youth football cannot be extrapolated from the high school, college, or professional experience. Injuries will occur in youth football because of the nature of the contact in the sport, and every effort should be made to reduce the injury risk.

References

[1]   Blyth, C. S. and Mueller, F. O., "Football Injury Survey: Part 1." *Physician Sportsmed,* Vol. 2, pp. 45–52.
[2]   Thompson, N., Halpern, B., Curl, W. et al. "High School Football Injuries: Evaluation," *American Journal of Sports Medicine,* Vol. 15, No. 2, 1987, pp. 117–124.
[3]   Powell, J., "636,000 Injuries Annually in High School Football," *Athletic Training,* Vol. 22, No. 1, 1991, pp. 19–22.
[4]   Nicholas, J. A., Rosenthal, P. P., Gleim, G. W., "A Historical Perspective of Injuries in Professional Football. Twenty-Six Years of Game-Related Events," *JAMA,* Vol. 4, No. 7, 1988, p. 260.
[5]   Zemper, E. D. "Injury Rates in a National Sample of College Football Teams: A 2-Year Prospective Sample," *Physician Sports Medicine,* Vol. 17, No. 11, 1989, pp. 100–113.
[6]   DeLee, J. C., Farney, W. C., Incidence of Injury in Texas High School Football, *American Journal of Sports Medicine,* Vol. No. 5, 1992, pp. ?.
[7]   Roser, L. A., Clawson, D. K., "Football Injuries in the Very Young Athlete," *Clinical Orthopedic Rel. Research,* Vol. 69, 1970, pp. 212–223.
[8]   Silverstein, B. M., "Injuries in Youth League Football," *Physician Sports Medicine* Vol. 7, No. 7, 1979, pp. 105–111.
[9]   Goldberg, B., Rosenthal, P., Nicholas, J. A., "Injuries in Youth Football," *Physician Sports Medicine,* Vol. 12, No. 8, 1984, pp. 122–131.
[10]   Goldberg, B., Rosenthal, P., Robertson, L., Nicholas, J., "Injuries in Youth Football," *Pediatrics,* Vol. 81, No. 2, 1988, pp. 255–261.

James P. Kelly, M.D.[1]

Head Injuries in Sports: Concussion Management in Football

REFERENCE: Kelly, J. P., "**Head Injuries in Sports: Concussion Management in Football,**" *Safety in American Football, ASTM STP 1305,* Earl F. Hoerner, Ed., American Society for Testing and Materials, 1996, pp. 35–41.

ABSTRACT: Surveys have found that 10% of college football players [1] and 20% of high school football players [2] experience concussions in a given football season. That translates to more than 250 000 concussions per year in football alone. The Sports Medicine Committee of the Colorado Medical Society drafted the "Guidelines for the Management of Concussion in Sports" that have subsequently been endorsed by several national physician organizations and widely distributed for the use of coaches, trainers, and allied health personnel as well as physicians. These guidelines are consistent with available evidence in clinical and research literature as well as consensus formed by medical experts.

KEYWORDS: concussion, contusion, return to play, tolerance, repeated trauma, observation continuing symptoms

Head injury in athletic and recreational activities is, unfortunately, a common occurrence. The most frequent head injury is that of concussion, defined as a traumatically induced alteration in mental status [3]. Certain sports are more prone to this problem, especially those contact or collision sports such as football, martial arts, and rugby. However, other forms of recreational or sports activities also carry some risk of traumatic brain injury such as horseback riding, ice hockey, and bicycling.

Information obtained from traumatic brain injury occurrences during organized athletic activities has taught us a great deal about how concussion occurs, what the individual experiences after concussion, and what the typical course of recovery is after such an injury. Unlike the majority of brain injuries in this country that result from motor vehicle collisions, falls, or assaults, those brain injuries that occur in organized sport activities are often witnessed and frequently captured on videotape or film. In many cases, a trained medical professional is available to examine the athlete and evaluate any worrisome neurological signs.

This information, combined with animal studies on the effects of traumatic brain injury has led to a growing body of medical and scientific literature on the subject [4,5]. Unfortunately, there are still widespread misconceptions about traumatic brain injury and its consequences. For instance, one can easily find textbooks and articles that define concussion as a brief loss of consciousness because of a blow to the head. It has been known for decades that concussion can occur without loss of consciousness [4,6,7]. In fact, most sports-related concussions occur without loss of consciousness. The true hallmarks of concussion are confusion and amnesia [3].

[1]Director, Brain Injury Program, Rehabilitation Institute of Chicago, 345 E. Superior St., Chicago, IL 60611, and assistant professor, Rehabilitation Medicine and Neurology, Northwestern University Medical School, 303 E. Chicago Avenue, Chicago, IL 60611.

Although it is true that the actual biomechanical threshold force necessary to produce brain injury has yet to be determined, there seems to be the agreement that forces applied in a rotational (angular) fashion are more likely to produce diffuse axonal injury, which is the anatomical change at the basis of concussion. These forces are often applied in combination with translational (linear) forces that tend to cause shifting of the brain inside the head, leading to contusions on the surface of the brain, further complicating the neurological condition [4]. In the years from 1984 to 1992, there have been 35 well-documented cases of incomplete recovery from cerebral injury in football alone [8].

There are two major considerations when looking at the athlete who has sustained a concussion. The first is that repeated concussions spaced near in time have been known to lead to catastrophic brain swelling that has been called the "second impact syndrome" [9]. This can lead to severe neurological disability or death. The athlete must be kept from risk of repeated concussion while still having symptomatic from the earlier concussion.

The second major concern is that of the well-documented cumulative effect of concussions [10] leading to persistent neurological abnormalities, postconcussion syndrome symptoms, and neuropsychological deterioration. Studies have shown that 25% of athletes with three concussions, 33% of those with four concussions, and 40% of those with five concussions showed persistent abnormalities on neuropsychological testing six months after their last injury [11]. Another review of concussion in football finds that the likelihood of concussion is six times greater for the athlete who has sustained a concussion within the last five years [12].

For many years, the Olympic Training Center in Colorado has been concerned that kicking at the head in martial arts is much more worrisome than most other athletic activities. In fact, a competitor in a Tai Kwan Do match is nearly eight times more likely to suffer a concussion than a player in a college football game [13].

The National Collegiate Athletic Association (NCAA) Injury Surveillance System reports the types of injuries for athletes in major college sports. Among those sports that require helmets, the incidence rate of concussion per "athlete-exposure" is highest in ice hockey, followed closely by football [14] (Table 1). Those sports that do not require head protection devices such as helmets are also associated with the risk of concussion. Men's and women's soccer lead the list, followed by field hockey and wrestling (Table 2). In most sports, these

TABLE 1—*Sports*[a] *with helmets.*

Sport	
Ice hockey	0.27
Football	0.25
Men's lacrosse	0.19
Women's softball	0.11

[a]Rate of concussions per 1000 athlete exposures.

TABLE 2—*Sports*[a] *without helmets.*

Sport	
Men's soccer	0.25
Women's soccer	0.24
Field hockey	0.20
Wrestling	0.20

[a]Rate of concussions per 1000 athlete exposures.

TABLE 3—*Features of concussion frequently observed.*

Features of Concussion

1	vacant stare,
2	delayed verbal and motor responses,
3	inability to focus attention,
4	disorientation,
5	slurred or incoherent speech,
6	gross observable incoordination or unsteady gait,
7	emotionality out of proportion to circumstances,
8	memory deficits, and
9	any period of loss of consciousness.

TABLE 4—*Common symptoms of concussion.*

Symptoms

Early:	
1	headache,
2	dizziness or vertigo,
3	lack of awareness of surroundings, and
4	nausea with or without vomiting.
Late:	
1	persistent low grade headache,
2	lightheadedness,
3	poor attention and concentration,
4	memory dysfunction,
5	excessive sleepiness or easy fatigue,
6	intolerance of bright lights or difficulty focusing vision,
7	intolerance of loud noises,
8	ringing in the ears,
9	anxiety and depressed mood, and
10	irritability and low frustration tolerance.

concussions are typically sustained by collisions among players [*14*]. A smaller percentage of concussions occur when the player's head strikes the ground or is struck by a ball, stick, or bat used in the sport. Some common features of concussion exhibited by athletes and symptoms they experience are listed in Tables 3 and 4, respectively. Symptoms that the athlete may experience are divided into "early" and "late" categories, although they may not confine themselves in all cases to a typical time course.

Concussion Management Guidelines

Members of the Colorado Medical Society published a report in 1990 after extensively reviewing the available medical literature and concluding that a new grading scale and management guideline for sports-related concussion should be created [*15*]. These "Colorado Guidelines" have subsequently been endorsed or adopted by several organizations (Table 5) and have been widely distributed for use by athletic trainers, allied health professionals, and physicians involved in the management of injured athletes. Coaches and athletes themselves should also become very familiar with these guidelines, recognizing concussion when it occurs and alerting healthcare professionals urgently [*16,17*].

TABLE 5—*Organizations endorsing or adopting the "Colorado guidelines."*

Organizations
American Academy of Pediatrics
American College of Surgeons—Committee on Trauma
American Academy of Sports Physicians
National Collegiate Athletic Association (NCAA)

The history of recent head trauma outside the sports setting, e.g., motor vehicle accident, should be considered in the "return to play" section for each grade of concussion (Table 6).

Grade 1—Confusion without amnesia, no loss of consciousness, and remove from event pending on-site evaluation prior to return.

This is the most common yet the most difficult form of concussion to recognize. The athlete is not rendered unconscious and suffers only momentary confusion. The majority of concussions in sports are of this type, and players commonly refer to it as having been "dinged" or having their "bell rung." All athletes with Grade 1 concussions should be removed from the game and evaluated before reentering the contest (Table 7).

Return to Play Following Grade 1 Concussion

Following a first Grade 1 concussion, if the athlete has no symptoms at rest or with exertion, return to the game may be permissible after at least 20 min of observation. In every instance when the athlete is symptomatic, removal from the game is mandatory. All symptoms (headache, dizziness, impaired orientation, impaired concentration, memory dysfunction) must have disappeared, first at rest and then with exertional provocative testing before return to competition (Table 7). Return is allowed only if the athlete is asymptomatic during rest and exertion for

TABLE 6—*Grading scale for concussion in sports.*

Grades for Concussion	
Grade 1	Confusion without amnesia, no loss of consciousness
Grade 2	Confusion with amnesia, no loss of consciousness, and
Grade 3	Loss of consciousness.

Guidelines for Return to Competition

Grade 1—Remove from contest. Examine immediately and every 5 min for the development of amnesia or postconcussive symptoms at rest and with exertion. (See Table 1). May return to contest if amnesia does not appear and no symptoms develop for at least 20 mins.

Grade 2—Remove from contest and do not allow return. Examine frequently for signs of evolving intracranial pathology. Reexamine the next day. May return to practice only after one full week without symptoms at rest and with exertion.

Grade 3—Transport from field by ambulance (with cervical spine immobilization if athlete remains unconscious) to nearest hospital. Thorough neurological evaluation immediately. Hospital confinement if signs of pathology are detected. If findings are normal, give instructions to family for overnight observation. May return to practice only after two full weeks without symptoms at rest and with exertion.

Symptoms—Prolonged unconsciousness, persistent mental status alterations, worsening postconcussion symptoms or abnormalities on neurological exam require urgent neurosurgical consultation or transfer to a trauma center.

TABLE 7—*Sideline evaluation.*

Mental Status Testing

Orientation: Time, place, person and situation (circumstances of injury)

Concentration: Digits backward
   3-1-7
   4-6-8-2
   5-9-3-7-4
   Months of year in reverse order

Memory: Names of teams in prior contest, President, Governor, Mayor; recent newsworthy events; three
   words and three objects at 0 and 5 min; details of contest (plays, moves, strategies, etc. as applicable)

Exertional Provocative Tests
   40 yd sprint,
   5 push-ups,
   5 sit-ups, and
   5 knee bends.
   (Any appearance of associated symptoms is abnormal, e.g., headache, dizziness, nausea, unsteadiness,
photophobia, blurred or double vision, emotional lability, or mental status changes.)

Neurological Tests
   Pupils: Symmetry and reaction,
   Coordination: Finger-nose-finger and tandem, and
   Sensation: Finger-nose (eyes closed) and Romberg.

at least 20 min. A second Grade 1 concussion in the same contest eliminates the player from competition that day. CT scanning or MRI scanning is recommended in all instances in which headache or other associated symptoms either worsen or persist longer than one week. It is recommended that three Grade 1 concussions terminate a player's season. No further contact sports are permitted for at least three months, and then only if asymptomatic at rest and with exertion.

Grade 2—Confusion with amnesia, no loss of consciousness, and remove from event and disallow return.

With a Grade 2 concussion, the athlete is not rendered unconscious but exhibits confusion and has amnesia for the events following the impact (posttraumatic amnesia). Amnesia for events preceding the injury (retrograde amnesia) may be seen along with posttraumatic amnesia in more severe cases. After a Grade 2 concussion, the athlete should be removed from the game and given a thorough neurological evaluation. The athlete should be evaluated frequently over the next 24 h for signs of evolving intracranial pathology by direct medical observation or with explicit, written instructions given to the family for monitoring the athlete at home.

Return to Play Following Grade 2 Concussion

Return to competition after a first concussion may be as soon as one week after the athlete is asymptomatic at rest and with exertion. A neurological exam should be performed by a physician before return to practice. CT scanning or MRI scanning is recommended in all instances in which headache or other associated symptoms either worsen or persist longer than one week. Return to contact play should be deferred for at least one month after a second Grade 2 concussion, and termination of the season should be considered. Terminating the season for that player is mandated by three Grade 2 concussions, as would by any abnormality on CT or MRI scan consistent with brain swelling, contusion, or other intracranial pathology.

Grade 3—Loss of consciousness, and remove from event and transport to appropriate medical facility.

It is usually quite easy to recognize a Grade 3 concussion. This level of head injury applies to any athlete who is rendered unconscious for any period of time. Initial treatment includes transport to the nearest hospital by ambulance, and the cervical spine should be immobilized if the athlete remains unconscious and cannot be fully evaluated. A thorough neurologic evaluation should be performed immediately. A neuroimaging study (CT or MRI scan) of the head should be performed in all athletes rendered unconscious even for brief periods of time. Hospital confinement is indicated if any signs of pathology are detected, or if the mental status of the athlete remains abnormal. If findings are normal, explicit written instructions may be given to the family for overnight observation. Neurological status should be assessed daily thereafter until all symptoms have resolved. The following are the symptoms to watch out for: Prolonged unconsciousness, persistent mental status alterations, worsening postconcussion symptoms, or abnormalities on neurological exam that require urgent neurosurgical consultation or transfer to a trauma center.

Return to Play Following Grade 3 Concussion

One month is the typical period the athlete should be held from contact sports after a Grade 3 concussion. Return to play before one month is allowed only if the athlete has been asymptomatic at rest and with exertion for at least two weeks. CT scanning or MRI scanning is recommended in all instances in which headache or other associated symptoms either worsen or persist longer than one week. A season is terminated by two Grade 3 concussions or by any abnormality on CT or MRI consistent with brain swelling, contusion, or other intracranial pathology. Return to any contact sport should be seriously discouraged in discussions with the athlete.

In most instances, when an athlete has suffered a head injury that requires intracranial surgery, return to contact sports is contraindicated. However, the final determination as to whether an athlete may return to competition is the team physician's clinical decision.

Conclusion

It is crucial that all individuals who participate in sports and recreational activities take into consideration the risk of traumatic brain injury and make every effort to prevent such potentially catastrophic problems. Physicians, athletic trainers, and coaches must become attuned to these problems and recognize even the mildest forms of concussion in athletes during practice or competition. It is essential that athletes themselves become well versed in the recognition and management of concussions so that they can participate in their own care from an informed perspective. We must all work more closely in breaking down barriers to the acceptance of concussion as a serious health problem. Our goal must be the elimination of this preventable neurologic disorder through education and prevention.

References

[1] Barth, J. T., Alves, W. M., Ryan, T. V., Macciocchi, S. N., Rimel, R. W., Jane, J. A. et al., "Mild Head Injury in Sports: Neuropsychological Sequelae and Recovery of Function," *Mild Head Injury,* H. S. Levin, H. M. Eisenberg, and A. L. Benton, Eds., Oxford University Press, New York, 1989, pp. 257–275.
[2] Gerberich, S. G., Priest, J. D., Boen, J. R., Straub, C. P., and Maxwell, R. E., "Concussion Incidence and Severity in Secondary School Varsity Football Players," *American Journal of Public Health,* Vol. 73, 1983, pp. 1370–1375.

[3] Kelly, J. P., Nichols, J. S., Filley, C. M., Lillehei, K. O., Rubinstein, D., and Kleinschmidt-DeMasters, B. K., "Concussion in Sports: Guidelines for the Prevention of Catastrophic Outcome," *Journal of the American Medical Association,* Vol. 266, No. 20, Nov. 1991, pp. 2867–2869.

[4] Ommaya, A. K. and Gennarelli, T. A., "Cerebral Concussion and Traumatic Unconsciousness: Correlation of Experimental and Clinical Observations on Blunt Head Injuries," *Brain,* Vol. 97, 1974, pp. 633–654.

[5] Povlishock, J. T. and Lontos, H. A., "Continuing Axonal and Vascular Change Following Experimental Brain Trauma," *Journal of Central Nervous System Trauma,* Vol. 2, 1985, pp. 285–298.

[6] Report of the Ad Hoc Committee to Study Head Injury Nomenclature: Proceedings of the Congress of Neurological Surgeons in 1964. *Clinical Neurosurgery,* Vol. 12, 1966, pp. 386–394.

[7] Fisher, C. M., "Concussion Amnesia," *Neurology,* Vol. 16, 1966, pp. 826–830.

[8] Mueller, F. O. and Cantu, R. C., "Annual Survey of Catastrophic Football Injuries: 1977–1992," *Head and Neck Injuries in Sports,* E. F. Hoerner, Ed., American Society for Testing and Materials, West Conshohocken, 1994, pp. 20–27.

[9] Saunders, R. L. and Harbaugh, R. E., "The Second Impact in Catastrophic Contact-Sports Head Trauma," *Journal of the American Medical Association,* Vol. 252, 1984, pp. 538–539.

[10] Gronwall, D. and Wrightson, P., "Cumulative Effect of Concussion," *Lancet,* Vol. 2, 1975, pp. 995–997.

[11] Leininger, B. E., Gramling, S. E., Fanell, H. D., Kreutzer, J. S., and Peck, E. A., "Neuropsychological Deficits in Symptomatic Minor Head Injury Patients After Concussion and Mild Concussion," *Journal of Neurology, Neurosurgery and Psychiatry,* Vol. 53, 1990, pp. 293–296.

[12] Zemper, E. D., "Analysis of Cerebral Concussion Frequency with the Most Commonly Used Models of Football Helmets," *Journal of Athletic Training,* Vol. 29, No. 1, 1994, pp. 44–50.

[13] Zemper, E. D. and Pieter, W., "Cerebral Concussions in Taekwondo Athletes," *Head and Neck Injuries in Sports,* E. F. Hoerner, Ed., American Society for Testing and Materials, West Conshohocken, 1994, pp. 116–123.

[14] Dick, R. W., "A Summary of Head and Neck Injuries in Collegiate Athletics Using the NCAA Injury Surveillance System," *Head and Neck Injuries in Sports,* E. F. Hoerner, Ed., American Society for Testing and Materials, West Conshohocken, 1994, pp. 13–19.

[15] Colorado Medical Society, "Report of the Sports Medicine Committee: Guidelines for the Management of Concussion in Sports," (revised), Colorado Medical Society, Denver, May, 1991.

[16] Kelly, J. P., "Concussion in Sports," *Current Therapy in Sports Medicine, 3rd Edition,* J. S. Torg and R. J. Shepard, Eds., Mosby, Philadelphia, 1995, pp. 21–24.

[17] M. T. Benson, Ed., "Guideline 20, Concussion and Second-Impact Syndrome," *1994–95 NCAA Sports Medicine Handbook,* The National Collegiate Athletic Association, Overland Park, KS, 1994, pp. 40–43.

Gerald A. Drake[1]

Catastrophic Football Injuries and Tackling Techniques

REFERENCE: Drake, G. A., "**Catastrophic Football Injuries and Tackling Techniques,**" *Safety in American Football, ASTM STP 1305,* Earl F. Hoerner, Ed., American Society for Testing and Materials, 1996, pp. 42–49.

ABSTRACT: The objective was to identify tackling techniques that contribute to cervical spinal cord injuries. First, the 19 tackles in the Prevent Paralysis II VHS documentary resulting in quadriplegia were analyzed for location, that is, above, at, or below the waist, direction, and head position, up or down. Second, records were kept for the same information on 3046 high school, college, and professional tackles during the 1993 season. Essentially, all tackles in the Prevent Paralysis II series were head down and resulted in quadriplegia. More than twice as many were below the waist rather than above the waist. Of the tackles below the waist, 83% were frontal and lateral at the level of the pelvis, thigh, or knee. Analysis of the 3046 tackles showed those below the waist were three times as likely to be head down, compared with tackles above the waist. Of the head down tackles below the waist, 83% were frontal or lateral at the level of the pelvis, thigh, or knee. It was concluded that head down tackling predisposes to cervical spine fracture/dislocations and spinal cord injury. The injury is most likely to occur when tackles are frontal and lateral at the level of the pelvis, thigh, and knee. Suggestions are to enforce penalties for head first contact and to establish rules that make tackling below the waist illegal except from behind, below the knee, and on initial contact in the existing 6 by 8 yd free blocking zone.

KEYWORDS: football, injuries, catastrophic, tackling, performance, incidence, risk factors

Since the 1976 rulings by the National Federation of State High School Associations and the National Collegiate Athletic Association rules committees to "get the head out of football," marked reductions in catastrophic and fatal injuries have occurred [1,2,4,5]. Yet during the last five seasons for which the data are available (1989–1993), an annual average of 2.4 high school football players have died from direct injuries (0.16/100 000) [2], and an annual average of 7.6 have suffered cervical spine fracture/dislocations resulting in spinal cord injury with incomplete recovery, some with permanent quadriplegia (0.51 per 100 000) [1].

There had been no direct college deaths for six years until one in 1994 [2]. An average of 0.8 college players per year have been left with unrecovered spinal cord injury (1.1 per 100 000) [1].

There have been no direct pro and semipro fatalities since 1972. During the past 15 years, one permanent cervical cord injury has occurred about every four years [1,2]. Rates per 100 000 are unknown.

From 1977 through 1993, a total of 167 catastrophic cervical cord injuries occurred. Of these, 70.6% were from tackling, 8.4% from being tackled, 3% from blocking, 5.4% from miscellaneous actions, and 12.6% were from unknown actions [1].

[1]Retired physician, M.D., 210-B Spring Lane, Chapel Hill, NC 27514. (Former member, Michigan State Medical Society Sports Medicine Committee.)

The 1993 Annual Survey of Football Injury Research says, "we must continue to reduce head and neck injuries" and "a continued effort should be made to keep the head out of the fundamental skills of football [2]." More specific measures may be needed to reduce further these tragic injuries. The research reported herein is a search for such measures. The research is based on the belief that "axial loading" of the cervical spine and consequent injuries, as described by Joseph Torg, are more likely to occur to the tackler when his head is down, which in turn is more likely to occur when tackles are below the waist. The following two questions are addressed:

1. Are cervical injuries in fact associated with head-down tackling?
2. Is the head down tackling position more likely to occur when the tackle is below the waist?

Answers to these questions may be helpful in enforcing and modifying current rules in a manner so as to reduce further the incidence of head and neck injuries in football.

Methods

Two methods were employed. First, the 19 tackles shown in the Prevent Paralysis II [3] VHS documentary were analyzed to determine the extent to which these injurious tackles were head down and below the waist. Second, records were kept during attendance at ten high school games and during viewing twelve college and sixteen professional games on television during the 1993 season. For 3046 tackles, notes were made on the location of the tackle, that is, whether it was above the waist, at the waist, or below the waist, and on the tackler's head position, up or down.

When the tackler's head was down, it appeared to be in the position described by Torg for axial loading of the cervical spine such that force impacted at the top of the helmet is transferred in a straight line through the spine [3,4,5]. Forward movement of the torso also increases the impact on the cervical spine. Such forces increase the risk of a fracture/dislocation resulting in spinal cord injury, possibly quadriplegia. Hitting with the head also increases the risk of serious or even fatal brain damage.

For tackles below the waist, records were made of whether they were from the front, the side, or behind and at what level (pelvis, thigh or knee versus below the knee). For about 20% of all tackles, it was impossible to determine the level and/or head position. They were excluded from the data.

Results

The Prevent Paralysis II VHS Documentary

Results of analysis of this documentary, covering 19 tackles that caused quadriplegia, are shown in Table 1 and Fig. 1. For some of the tackles, it was difficult to determine the level and head position at the instant of the damaging impact, but a trend was apparent. Essentially, all tackles appeared to be head down except for possibly two head-to-head impacts which were angled such that considerable force had to be delivered to the cervical spine. More than twice as many tackles resulting in quadriplegia were below the waist rather than above the waist. Specifically, 26% were above the waist, 11% were at the waist, and 63% were below the waist ($p < 0.02$).

Of the tackles below the waist, 83% were frontal or lateral at the level of the pelvis, thigh or knee, and 17% were below the knee ($p < 0.021$). None were from behind.

TABLE 1—*Analysis of Prevent Paralysis II video (tackles causing quadriplegia, all essentially head down).*

Parameters	Frequency	Percent
Tackles Above the Waist	5[a]	26
Tackles at the Waist	2	11
Tackles Below the Waist	12[b]	63
Total	19	100
Chi-square $= 8.316$; $p < 0.02$		
Breakdown of Tackles below the Waist		
Frontal & Lateral Pelvis, Thigh, and Knee	10	83
Below Knee	2[b]	17
Total	12	100
Chi-square $= 5.333$; $p < 0.021$		

[a]Two of these were head-to-head hits with head position indeterminate.
[b]One of these was an attempted fumble recovery rather than a tackle.

In summary, analysis of the documentary shows that a high percentage of paralysis-causing tackles are below the waist, either frontal or lateral, and with the head down.

High School Tackles

Results from the analysis of 809 high school tackles are shown in Fig. 2. Of the tackles above the waist, 3% were head down; of the tackles at the waist, 6% were head down; and of the tackles below the waist, 13% were head down ($p < 0.001$). Four times as many tackles below the waist were head down compared to tackles above the waist.

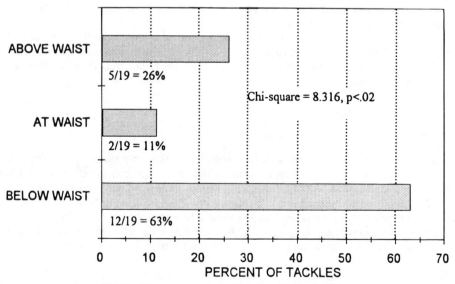

FIG. 1—*Prevent paralysis II series—level of tackles.*

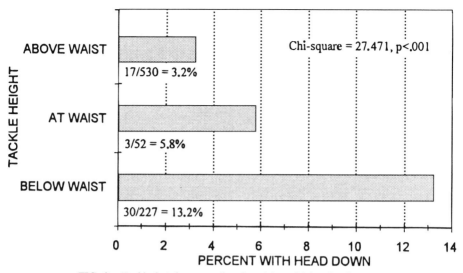

FIG. 2—*Tackle height versus head position—high school games.*

College Tackles

Results from the analysis of 1160 college tackles are shown in Fig. 3. Of the tackles above the waist, 5% were head down; of the tackles at the waist, 8% were head down; and of the tackles below the waist, 14% were head down ($p < 0.001$).

Professional Tackles

Results from the analysis of 1077 professional tackles are shown in Fig. 4. Of the tackles above the waist, 4% were head down; of the tackles at the waist, 8% were head down; and of the tackles below the waist, 12% were head down ($p < 0.001$).

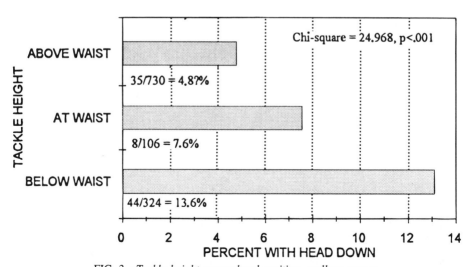

FIG. 3—*Tackle height versus head position—college games.*

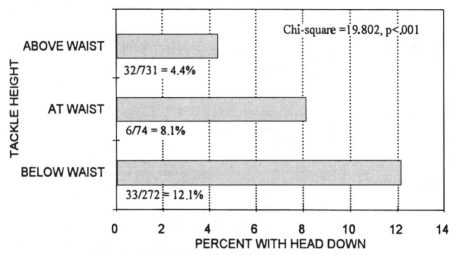

FIG. 4—*Tackle height versus head position—pro games.*

Combined High School, College, and Professional

Results from the combined analysis of 3046 high school, college, and professional tackles are shown in Table 2 and summarized in Fig. 5. Of the tackles above the waist, 4% were head

TABLE 2—*Tackle height and head position in high school, college & pro games.*

Type of Tackle	Frequencies				Percentages			
	High School	College	Pro	All	High School	College	Pro	All
All Tackles	1113	1402	1293	3808	100	100	100	100
Unanalyzable Tackles	304	242	216	762	27	17	17	20
Analyzable Tackles	809	1160	1077	3046	73	83	83	80
Above Waist	530	730	731	1991	66	63	68	65
Head up	513	695	699	1907	97	95	96	96
Head down	17	35	32	84	3	5	4	4
At Waist	52	106	74	232	6	9	7	8
Head up	49	98	68	215	94	92	92	93
Head down	3	8	6	17	6	8	8	7
Below Waist	227	324	272	823	28	28	25	27
Head up	197	280	239	716	87	86	88	87
Head down	30	44	33	107	13	14	12	13
Breakdown of Below Waist								
Pelvis Through Knee	152	206	170	528	67	64	63	64
Front and Side	77	128	101	306	51	62	59	58
Head up	53	89	75	217	69	70	74	71
Head down	24	39	26	89	31	30	26	29
Behind	75	78	69	222	49	38	41	42
Head up	74	76	66	216	99	97	96	97
Head down	1	2	3	6	1	3	4	3
Below Knee	75	118	102	295	33	36	38	36
Head up	70	115	98	283	93	97	96	96
Head down	5	3	4	12	7	3	4	4

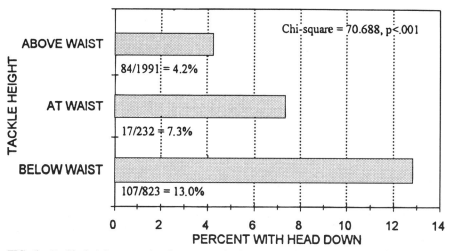

FIG. 5—*Tackle height versus head position—high school, college and pro games combined.*

down; of the tackles at the waist, 7% were head down; and of the tackles below the waist, 13% were head down ($p < 0.001$). Compared to tackling above the waist, tackling below the waist is three times as likely to put the head down and the cervical spine at risk of injury.

Of the combined 3046 tackles, 65% were above the waist, 8% were at the waist, and 27% were below the waist. This was consistent within 3% for all three groups.

A breakdown of all 823 tackles below the waist is shown in Fig. 6. This analysis shows that tacklers are more likely to put their heads down when tackling from the front and side below the waist. Of 306 tackles at the frontal and lateral aspects of the pelvis, thigh and knee, 71% were head up and 29% were head down. For tackles from behind at the same level, of

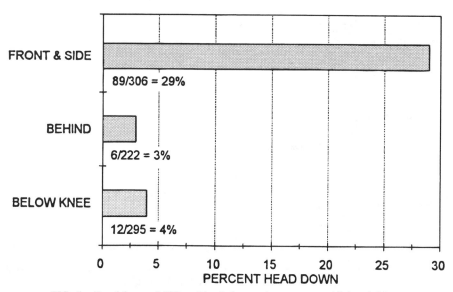

FIG. 6—*Breakdown of 823 tackles below waist—percent with head down.*

222 such tackles, 97% were head up and 3% were head down. For tackles below the knees, of 295 such tackles, 96% were head up and 4% were head down.

Figure 7 shows that of the 107 head down tackles below the waist 83% were from the front and side at the pelvis, thigh and knee levels, 6% were from behind and 11% were below the knee.

In summary, for all tackles above the waist there was one chance in 25 a tackle would be head down. For tackles below the waist, the chance was one in eight it would be head down, and for frontal and lateral tackles at the level of the pelvis, thigh, and knee, the chance was one in three.

Discussion

The first question addressed in this report is whether cervical injuries are associated with head down tackling. Analysis of the Prevent Paralysis II documentary shows that almost two-thirds of the tackles resulting in quadriplegia were below the waist with the head down. The remaining tackles in the video were at or above the waist with the head essentially down. Clearly, head down tackling puts the tackler at risk.

The second question is whether the head down tackling position is more likely to occur when the tackle is below the waist. Analysis of high school, college, and professional tackles shows that when tackling below the waist, the tackler is three times as likely to put his head down, putting his head and cervical spine at risk.

It is clear that head down tackling is dangerous and that tackling below the waist increases head down tackling. Can more be done to prevent the occurrence of this dangerous practice? Although data on officiating were not included in this study, it is true that in the games observed, penalties for head first contact, whether tackling or carrying the ball, were seldom called. The Annual Survey of Catastrophic Football Injuries says, "The use of the helmet-face mask in making initial contact while blocking and tackling is illegal and should be called for

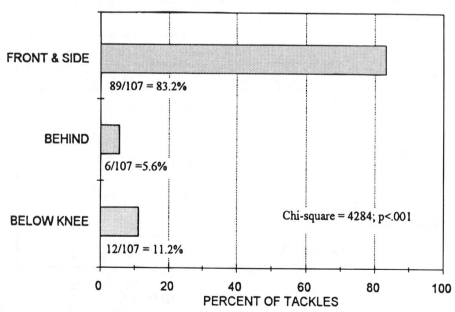

FIG. 7—*Direction of head down tackles below waist.*

a penalty . . . If more of these penalties are called, there is no doubt that players and coaches will get the message and discontinue this type of play [1]."

Suggestions

The following suggestions are offered for consideration as a means of further reducing the incidence of serious head and cervical spinal injuries in football:

(1) Enforce penalties for head first contact.
(2) Establish penalties that make below the waist tackling illegal except from behind, below the knees, and on initial contact in the existing 6 by 8 yd free blocking zone for tacklers in that zone when play starts. (Note that rules limiting blocking below the waist are now enforced to prevent knee and ankle injuries. Surely, prevention of much more tragic, even if much rarer, head and neck injuries justifies similar rule changes for tackling and ball carrying.)
(3) Encourage game officials to review Prevent Paralysis II and use the depicted tackles as models for calling penalties.
(4) Encourage all participants in organized football, including coaching staffs, players, and the parents of players who are minors, to view Prevent Paralysis II.

Although these changes might favor the offense, a 33 to 30 game is more exciting than a 3 to 0 game. Infinitely more important, these changes could help attain the ultimate goal of eliminating fatal and catastrophic football injuries.

References

[1] Mueller, F. O. and Cantu, R. C., "Annual Survey of Catastrophic Football Injuries, 1977–1993," Unpublished manuscript.
[2] Mueller, F. O. and Schindler, R. D., "Annual Survey of Football Injury Research, 1931–1993," Report submitted to the American Football Coaches Association, Feb. 1993.
[3] Prevent Paralysis II. 11 minute VHS documentary produced by J. Torg, et al. at the University of Pennsylvania Sports Medicine Center (235 S. 33rd St., Philadelphia, PA 19104), and the National Federation of State High School Associations with a grant from Riddell, Inc.
[4] Torg, J. S., Truex, R., Jr., Quedenfeld, T. C., et al., "The National Football Head and Neck Injury Registry Report and Conclusions 1978," *Journal of the American Medical Association,* Vol. 241, 1979, pp. 1477–1479.
[5] Torg, J. S., Vegso, J. J., O'Neill, M. J., et al., "The Epidemiologic, Pathologic, Biomechanical, and Cinematographic Analysis of Football-Induced Cervical Spine Trauma," *American Journal of Sports Medicine,* Vol. 18, 1990, pp. 50–57.

Science

Robert C. Cantu[1]

Guidelines for Return to Contact Sports After Transient Quadriplegia

REFERENCE: Cantu, R. C., "**Guidelines for Return to Contact Sports After Transient Quadriplegia,**" *Safety in American Football, ASTM STP 1305,* Earl F. Hoerner, Ed., American Society for Testing and Materials, 1996, pp. 53–59.

ABSTRACT: Three cases seen by the author will be presented that illustrate acceptable circumstances, as well as relative and absolute contraindications for athletes to return to contact/collision sports after an incident of transient quadriplegia. Return is deemed acceptable if the athlete has complete resolution of symptoms, full range of motion, and normal curvature of the cervical spine, as well as no evidence of spinal stenosis on magnetic resonance (MR) imaging, contrast enhanced computerized tomography (CT), or myelography. Relative contraindications, as seen in Case 2, involve a mild intervertebral disc bulge that does not obliterate the reserve of cerebrospinal fluid (CSF) around the cord and transient quadriplegia caused by minimal contact. In Case 3, true spinal stenosis documented by MR imaging illustrates an absolute contraindication for return to contact/collision sports after an episode of transient quadriplegia and what can happen if return is allowed. The author realizes that these guidelines would be difficult to prove in a scientific fashion, and that the legal and moral consequences of a controlled trial would be too serious to allow it to be done.

KEYWORDS: stenosis, stingers, return to play, catastrophic injury, assessment, quadriplegia

Before the advent of computed tomography (CT) and, more recently, magnetic resonance imaging (MR) scanning, the presence of cervical spinal stenosis was defined by bony measurements. In 1956, Wolf et al. [1], using randomly selected asymptomatic subjects who underwent lateral cervical spine radiographs at a fixed target distance of 72 in. (183 cm) to eliminate magnification error, established normal values of the sagittal diameters of the cervical spine. Sagittal diameter canal height was defined as the anteroposterior diameter measured from the posterior aspect of the vertebral body to the most anterior point on the spinolaminar line. Wolfe and colleagues found the average anteroposterior diameter was 22 mm at C-1, 20 mm at C-2, and 17 mm from C-3 to C-7 [1]. General consensus evolved in the radiologic literature that between C-3 and C-7 when magnification is corrected for that canal heights are normal above 15 mm [2,3] and spinal stenosis is present below 13 mm [4,5].

In 1986, Torg et al. [6] and, in 1987, Pavlov et al. [7], described a new method to assess cervical spinal stenosis radiographically using a ratio method to eliminate the need to correct radiographic magnification error. The height of the spinal canal, as measured from the midpoint of the posterior surface of the vertebral body up to the spinolaminar line, is the numerator, and the denominator is the height of the corresponding midvertebral body. A vertebral canal/vertebral body ratio of less than 0.80 was defined as "significant spinal stenosis."

---

[1]Director, Chief Neurosurgery Service, Service of Sports Medicine, Emerson Hospital, Concord MA 01742.

Recently, the Torg ratio, as a means to define spinal stenosis, has been cast in doubt. First, the Kerlan Jobe Orthopedic Clinic found the incidence of spinal stenosis using the Torg "ratio" to be 33% in 124 professional and 100 rookie football players [8].

More recently, Herzog et al. [9] found in 80 asymptomatic professional football players that 49% had abnormal ratios below 0.80 at one or more cervical levels. They also found the ratio to be highly unreliable in determining spinal stenosis with a positive predictive value of only 12%. They found that their athletes had normal canal heights (numerator) but often massive vertebral bodies (denominator), which brought the ratio to less than 0.80. They concluded "if an abnormal Torg ratio is detected, further evaluation is necessary before an athlete can be diagnosed as significantly spinal stenotic" [9].

More recently, I have proposed [10,11] that currently only diagnostic technologies that view the spinal cord itself, such as MRI, contrast-positive CT (CT+), or myelography, should be used to establish the diagnosis of cervical spinal stenosis. Only these technologies and not an X ray or X ray ratio assess the size of the neural tissue in relation to the size of the spinal canal. The size of the cervical spinal cord, although usually 9 to 10 mm in diameter, has been reported to vary between 4 and 11.5 mm [12,13]. Thus, true stenosis may be present with low to normal canal measurements and a large spinal cord.

I have also advanced the concept of "functional spinal stenosis" [14,15] as defined by the loss of the "functional reserve" of cerebrospinal fluid (CSF) around the cord, or actual deformation of the spinal cord. Only the MRI, CT+ or myelogram clearly shows whether the spinal cord has a normal functional reserve: the space around the cord largely filled with a protective cushion of cerebrospinal fluid between the cord and the spinal canal's interior walls lined by bone, disc, and ligament. In addition, these technologies can also determine whether the spinal cord is deformed by an abnormality such as disc protrusion or rupture, bony osteophyte, or posterior buckling of the ligamentus flavum.

Return-to-Play Criteria for Contact or Collision Sports After Cervical Spine or Cord Injury

Sprain or Strain

Most cervical injuries will involve a ligament sprain, muscle strain, or contusion. With such injuries, there is no neurological or osseous injury, and return to competition can occur when the athlete is free of neck pain with and without axial compression, range of motion is full, and the strength of the neck is normal. Cervical X rays should show no subluxation or abnormal curvatures. If the athlete has a neck profile or maximal weight that he or she can pull with the neck in flexion, extension, and to each side, it is preferable the athlete not return to competition until he or she is asymptomatic, and can perform to the level of his or her preinjury profile.

Cervical Spine Fracture

Stable fractures that have healed completely will allow the player to return by the next season. If there is a one-level anterior or posterior fusion for a fracture, athletes are usually allowed to go back when the neck pain is gone, the range of motion is complete, muscle strength of the neck is normal, and the fusion is solid. In any athlete with a fractured neck, proper warnings against contact or collision sports are advisable until it is certain that the patient is completely healed.

Where there are multilevel fusions or a fusion involving C1-2 or C2-3, return to contact collision sports is contraindicated, but the athlete could participate in a noncontact sport at low risk of neck injury such as tennis.

Return-to-Play Criteria After a Burner

Roughly, half of so-called "burners" or "stingers" in football at the high school level involve a brachial plexus stretch injury. The majority at the college and professional level involve a cervical nerve root "pinch" phenomenon within the neural foramen. Because the dorsal root ganglion occupies most of the space with the foramen and lies underneath the subluxing facet, it often takes the brunt of the injury, and symptoms may be purely sensory in a dermatomal distribution. This is especially true if the athlete has had similar symptoms before. If there are any residual symptoms, or neck pain, or incomplete range of motion, or suspicion of a neck injury, return should be deferred.

Return-to-Play Criteria After Transient Quadriplegia

What factors predispose athletes to quadriplegia and when should athletes be withheld from future participation in contact or collision sports after an episode of transient quadriplegia? What are the appropriate circumstances to allow return after transient quadriplegia and what are *relative* and *absolute* contraindications for return? In presenting and discussing three case histories seen in my practice, these questions will be answered.

Case Histories

Case 1 involved a 27-year-old National Football League linebacker who experienced transient upper and lower extremity paralysis and numbness after tackling a 225-lb (102-kg) opponent. The patient made contact sufficient to dent the forehead portion of his helmet and appeared to sustain an axial load injury with some hyperextension. Paralysis lasted 4 min, then, over the next 10 to 20 min, motor and sensory function returned beginning in the lower extremities. On arrival at the hospital, the patient was complaining of a burning sensation across his neck and shoulders. He denied any loss of consciousness, and there was no loss of bowel or bladder function.

On physical examination, higher cortical functions were intact. Motor examination results were 5/5 throughout, and reflexes were 2+ and symmetric except the ankles, which were 1+ and symmetric. Plantar response was downgoing bilaterally. Sensory examination results were positive to light touch and pinprick. The cerebellum was intact on examination.

Plain films of the cervical spine showed no evidence of fracture, dislocation, or subluxation, or degenerative disc disease. The canal height measured within normal limits: 15 mm at C-3 and C-4 and 20 mm at C-6. Torg ratios were C-3 = 15/24 = 0.63, C-4 = 15/22 = 0.68, C-5 = 17/20 = 0.85, C-6 = 20/22 = 0/91. MRI showed no evidence of fracture, canal compromise, or contusion. Flexion and extension views of the spine showed no instability. Cervical CT and MRI showed a functional reserve of CSF around the cord.

Case 2 involved a 23-year-old hockey player, drafted into the National Hockey League, who was injured while filming a team advertisement. Bending at the waist with his neck flexed, he unexpectedly collided with another player. The top of the patient's helmet struck the other player's abdomen. The patient's neck was relaxed because he was not expecting impact. Each player had taken one stride before the impact. The patient had immediate neck pain and felt something was wrong with his arms and legs. He fell to his side and rolled over on the ice onto his back. After 1 min, he was aware that he could move his fingers in his gloves and his toes in his skates. A pins-and-needles sensation extended into both hands and, to a lesser extent, his torso and legs. He was aware of a rigid painful neck within minutes. When he moved his head, a shocklike sensation traveled down his spine to his buttocks. It was about 4 or 5 min before he could rise from the ice. Neurological symptoms persisted at highest intensity for approximately 5 min, then gradually subsided, first in his legs and then his arms. It was two weeks before all paresthesias disappeared. Other than a brief concussion in 1984, when his helmeted head struck the boards, he denied any significant prior injury.

Two weeks after injury, the patient had normal range of neck motion. No radiating symptoms could be elicited by compression of his spinous processes or by mild axial loading (negative Spurling's maneuver). No neurologic deficit was detected. Strength and tone were normal throughout. Plantar responses were downgoing. No clonus or abnormal reflexes were present. Upper extremity reflexes were 1+ and lower extremity reflexes were 2+. Gait proved normal and no sensory loss for pinprick, vibration, or position sense was found.

Plain films showed no evidence of degenerative disc disease, subluxation, or fracture. The height of the canal at all levels exceeded 15 mm. Torg ratios measured C-3 = 17/24 = −0.71; C-4 = 15/23 = 0.65; C-5 = 15/26 = 0.68; C-6 = 16/23 = 0.70. MRI revealed mild disc bulging at C3-4 but did not show spinal cord encroachment, and did show a functional reserve of CSF around the cord at all levels. Myelogram and CT+ showed slight disc bulging at C3-4 but also CSF around the spinal cord at all levels, including C3-4.

The athlete in Case 3 first injured his neck as a high school football player in 1987. Upon making what he remembers to be a head-up tackle, he fell to his side and was unable to get up or roll onto his back. Sensation and motor movement were absent from the neck down. Gradually, motor function and sensation returned, first in his feet and then his hands. He could not move his head because of cervical spasm, and any attempts to do so produced jabs of pain running from his neck to his head. After several minutes, he was able to stand and walk off the field unassisted, although his legs felt very weak. His neck was rigid on the sidelines and he did not return to play. No X rays were taken at that time and no medical attention was sought. The patient played the following week with a neck collar. He reported that his neck was rigid and thus he performed poorly. He did not play for the next two weeks because of continued rigidity and severe neck pain. Three weeks after the injury, because of persistent neck pain and stiffness, he sought medical attention at a sports medicine facility. There, cervical spine X rays were taken. Although canal heights and Torg ratios were not measured, subsequent review of these films revealed canal heights of 12 mm consistent with spinal stenosis and abnormal Torg ratios at C-4 = 12/25 = 0.48, and C-5 = 12/24 = 0.50. After two weeks, the patient returned to competition, his neck pain and stiffness relieved. He played his senior season without further cervical symptoms.

The following fall, as a college freshman on full athletic scholarship, the patient squatted to make a tackle, hitting face to face and chest to chest. With head tilted up, his facemask made first contact. He fell backward on the ground, unable to move and without sensation from the neck down. Over the next few minutes, movement began to return to his right side and patchy sensation to his left side. He was transported to the hospital where physical examination showed cranial nerves to be intact. There was a Brown-Sequard syndrome with right-sided hemisensory loss and a nearly flaccid left side. Muscle strength was 4/5 on the right except the intrinsic muscles of the hand, which were 3/5. Biceps reflex are 1+ and symmetric, triceps reflex was 2 pl on the right and absent on the left, knee jerk reflex was 2+ on the right and absent on the left, ankle jerk reflex was 2+ on the right and 1+ on the left. There were three beats of clonus in both ankles.

X rays, CTs, and MRIs were taken. The films revealed cervical stenosis and posterior disc herniation at C-3 and C-4 with displacement of cord and thecal sac to the right. Torg ratios measured C-2 = 20/23 = 0.87; C-3 = 13/23 = 0.52; C-5 = 12/24 = 0.50; C-6 and C-7 could not be read. Edema was found within the spinal cord from C-2 to C-5. Surgery was performed without complications, but the patient remained paralyzed immediately afterward. A second exploration did not find bleeding. The patient went to rehabilitation and remained in a wheelchair for eight months before walking. Presently, he has recovered to a spastic quadriparetic state.

Discussion

All three athletes in these cases suffered a bout of transient quadriplegia. Although such an event may occur after hyperextension or hyperflexion, it most frequently occurs with axial load injury to the cervical spine, as described by Torg [6]. In all cases, the symptoms were consistent with variations of the central spinal cord syndrome as described by Schneider et al. [16].

Cervical spinal stenosis is known to increase the risk of permanent neurological injury [17–19]. Firooznia et al. [20] presented three case reports of patients who became quadriplegic after only "minor trauma." In all three patients, radiological studies revealed "marked stenosis of the spinal canal." Some debate exists, however, over the definition of spinal stenosis. In the past, the anteroposterior (AP) diameter of the spinal canal, measured from the posterior aspect of the vertebral body to the most anterior point on the spinolaminar line, determined the presence of stenosis. General consensus has been that between C-3 and C-7, canal heights are normal above 15 mm and spinal stenosis is present below 13 mm [1]. Resnick says CT and myelography are "the most sensitive diagnostic modalities" in determining spinal stenosis [21]. He points out that roentgenography fails to appraise the width of the cord, and is not useful when stenosis results from ligamentous hypertrophy or discal protrusion. Ladd and Scranton [5] state that the AP diameter of the spinal canal is "unimportant" if there is total impedance of the contrast medium. They argue that metrizamide-enhanced myelogram is needed for the injured athlete because CT alone fails to reveal neural compression adequately. Thus, spinal stenosis cannot be defined by bony measurements alone. "Functional" spinal stenosis, defined as loss of the CSF around the cord or, in more extreme cases (i.e., Case 3), deformation of the spinal cord, whether documented by CT+, MRI, or myelography, is a more accurate measure of stenosis [10]. The term "functional" is taken from the radiological term "functional reserve" as applied to the protective cushion of CSF around the spinal cord in a nonstenotic canal [9]. In a recent study in which MRI was used to document the presence or absence of spinal stenosis in 11 athletes rendered quadriplegic, six had functional stenosis [10]. Furthermore, in the data from the National Center for Catastrophic Sports Injury Research, cases of quadriplegia without spine fracture have been seen only when functional spinal stenosis is present. Also, complete recovery of neurological function after initial neurological deficit after spine fracture or dislocation has been seen only in the absence of functional spinal stenosis.

Of the three athletes presented, only Case 3 was documented as having cervical spinal stenosis as determined by AP diameter alone (12 mm at C-4 and C-5). In both Cases 1 and 2, the narrowest AP diameter measured 15 mm. In Case 1, CT and MRI showed no abnormalities and did show a functional reserve of CSF around all levels of the cord. In Case 2, CT, MRI, and myelogram all showed slight disc bulging at C3-4, but again showed a reserve of CSF around the cord at all levels. After the second injury, in Case 3, the patient was shown to suffer functional cervical spinal stenosis. CT and MRI also showed spinal cord edema and displacement of the cord secondary to disc herniation.

Torg ratios were abnormal for all three athletes, with minimum ratios of 0.63 for Case 1, 0.65 for Case 2, and 0.40 for Case 3. This ratio (canal height/vertebral body AP diameter) of less than 0.80 has been defined as spinal stenosis [3]. For Cases 1 and 2, this ratio is misleading because the large vertebral body, not a narrow canal, produced ratios less than 0.80. This is consistent with other reports that an abnormal Torg ratio is a poor predictor of true functional stenosis [9]. Although the ratio leads to many false-positive results (positive predictive value at 12%) [9], it rarely is normal when true stenosis documented by MRI is present (sensitivity = 92%) [9]. Thus, an abnormal ratio in an athlete with spinal cord symptoms means that evaluation with MRI, myelogram, or CT+ should be done.

Given an athlete who has suffered transient quadriplegia, what criteria should be followed for his or her return to contact sports? Case 1 is an example of an athlete who has never had these symptoms. This athlete had complete neurological recovery and full range of cervical spine movement. AP diameter was normal at all levels; CT and MRI showed no evidence of functional stenosis. Thus, there were no neurological, mechanical, symptomatic, or structural (functional spinal stenosis) contraindications for return to competition. Understanding that he may be at slightly greater risk for a second event, the athlete returned to competition and has had no further symptoms.

Case 2 involved an athlete who has two relative contraindications for returning to play, namely, mild disc bulging at C3-4, and the fact that the impact that produced the transient quadriplegia seemed relatively minor (head-to-abdomen contact from one step apart). Because myelogram and CT did not show functional stenosis and his cervical strength and range of motion returned to normal, there was not an absolute contraindication to return to play. After consideration of the relative contraindications, this athlete chose not to return to professional hockey.

Case 3 is an example of an athlete with an absolute contraindication for return. In addition to a stenotic canal according to AP diameter (12 mm), he had functional stenosis on CT and MRI with cord displacement, edema and lack of reserve CSF around the cord at all levels secondary to disc herniation. Because studies were not performed after his initial injury, it is not known whether he had a cord displacement at that time, but the stenosis was present. This should have been evaluated by MRI, myelogram, or CT+, and the presence of functional stenosis should have terminated his football career after the initial episode of transient quadriplegia. If he had not had severe spinal stenosis, it is probable his subsequent disc herniation would have produced radicular symptoms alone instead of severe spinal cord injury.

Given an athlete with cervical spinal stenosis, what is the mechanism of injury causing transient or permanent neurologic deficit? Eismont et al. [22] state that such athletes are "remarkably susceptible to hyperextension injuries known to produce maximal narrowing (up to 2 mm) of the ventrodorsal diameter of the spinal canal." Torg and others [5] note that hyperextension causes "an inward indentation of the ligamentum flavum," which can compress the cord. Penning [23] described a "bony pincers" mechanism in hypoextension in which the cord is compressed between the vertebral body and the closest portion of the spinolaminar line of the inferior vertebra. The athlete in Case 3 appeared to suffer a hyperextension injury making contact with the facemask, and it was spinal stenosis that predisposed him to neurological injury. The athletes in Cases 1 and 2 suffered axial load injuries. The blow in Case 1 was severe enough to dent the helmet. In Case 2, although the force of the blow was not great, the contact was not expected and therefore the athlete's neck muscles were relaxed, causing greater transmission of forces directly on the spine instead of being dissipated in the muscles.

Conclusion

These three athletes present a spectrum of when to allow return to competition in contact or collision sports after an episode of transient quadriplegia. It is important to realize that normal canal size on lateral X-ray does not preclude the possibility of functional spinal stenosis—an absolute contraindication for return. For this diagnosis, myelogram, CT+, or MRI is needed.

References

[1] Wolfe, B. S., Khilnani, M., and Malis, L., "The Sagittal Diameter of the Bony Cervical Spinal Canal and Its Significance in Cervical Spondylosis," *Journal of the Mount Sinai Hospital*, Vol. 23, 1956, pp. 283–292.

[2]   Alexander, M. M., Davis, C. H., and Field, C. H., "Hyperextension Injuries of the Cervical Spine," *Archives of Neurology and Psychiatry*, Vol. 79, 1958, pp. 146–150.
[3]   Boijsen, E. "The Cervical Spinal Canal in Intraspinal Expansive Processes," *Acta Radiologica*, Vol. 42, 1954, pp. 101–115.
[4]   Epstein, J. A., Carras, R., Hyman, R. A., et al., "Cervical Myelopathy Caused by Developmental Stenosis of the Spinal Canal." *Journal of Neurosurgery*, Vol. 51, 1979, pp. 362–367.
[5]   Ladd, A. L. and Scranton, P. E., "Congenital Cervical Stenosis Presenting as Transient Quadriplegia in Athletes," *Journal of Bone and Joint Surgery*, Vol. 68, 1986, pp. 1371–1374.
[6]   Torg, J. S., Pavlov, H., Genuano, S. E., et al., "Neuropraxia of the Cervical Spinal Cord with Transient Quadriplegia," *Journal of Bone and Joint Surgery*, Vol. 68A, 1986, pp. 1354–1378.
[7]   Pavlov, H., Torg, J. S., Robie, B., et al., "Cervical Spinal Stenosis: Determination with Vertebral Body Ratio Method," *Radiology*, Vol. 164, 1987, pp 771–775.
[8]   Odor, J. M., Watkins, R. G., Dillin, W. H., Dennis, S., and Saberi, M., Incidence of Cervical Spinal Stenosis in Professional and Rookie Football Players, *American Journal of Sports Medicine*, Vol. 18, 1990, pp. 507–509.
[9]   Herzog, R. J., Weins, J. J., Dillingham, M. F., and Sontag, M. J., "Normal Cervical Spine Morphometry and Cervical Spinal Stenosis in Asymptomatic Professional Football Players," *Spine*, Vol. 16, 1991, pp. 178–186.
[10] Cantu, R. C., Functional cervical spinal stenosis: a contraindication to participation in contact sports. *Medicine and Sciences in Sports and Exercise*, Vol. 25, 1993.
[11] Cantu, R. V. and Cantu, R. C., "Guidelines for Return to Contact Sports after Transient Quadriplegia." *Journal of Neurosurgery*, Vol. 80, 1994, pp. 592–594.
[12] Lamont, A. C., Zachary, J., and Sheldon, P. W., "Cervical Cord Size in Metrizamide Myelography," *Clinical Radiology*, Vol. 32, 1981, pp. 409–412.
[13] Thijssen, H. O., Keyser, A., Horstink, M. W., et al., "Morphology of the Cervical Spinal Cord on Computed Myelography," *Neuroradiology*, Vol. 18, 1979, pp. 57–62.
[14] Cantu, R. C., Letter to the editor. *Medicine and Science in Sports and Exercise*, Vol. 25, 1993, pp. 1082–1084.
[15] Cantu, R. C., "Cervical Spinal Stenosis: Challenging an Established Detection Method," *Physician and Sports Medicine*, Vol. 21, 1993, pp. 57–63.
[16] Schneider, R. S., Reifel, E., Crisler, H., et al., "Serious and Fatal Football Injuries Involving the Head and Spinal Cord," *Journal of American Medical Association*, Vol. 177, 1961, pp. 362–367.
[17] Matsuura, P., Waters, R. L., Adkins, R. H., Rothman, S., Gurbani, W., and Sie, I., "Comparison of Computerized Tomography Parameters of the Cervical Spine in Normal Control Subjects and Spinal Cord-Injured Patients," *Journal of Bone and Joint Surgery*, Vol. 71, 1989, pp. 183–188.
[18] Mayfield, F. H., "Neurosurgical Aspects of Cervical Trauma," *Clinical Neurosurgery, Vol. II*, Baltimore: Williams & Wilkins, 1955.
[19] Nugent, G. R., "Clinicopathologic Correlations in Cervical Spondylosis," *Neurology*, Vol. 9, 1959, pp. 273–281.
[20] Firooznia, H., Ahn, J., Rafii, M., et al., "Sudden Quadriplegia after a Minor Trauma. The Role of Pre-Existing Spinal Stenosis," *Surgical Neurology*, Vol. 23, 1985, pp. 165–168.
[21] Resnick, D., "Degenerative Disease of the Spine," *Diagnosis of Bone and Joint Disorders*, New York: W. B. Saunders Co., 1981, pp. 1408–1415.
[22] Eismont, F. J., Clifford, S., Goldberg, M., et al., "Cervical Sagittal Spinal Canal Size in Spinal Injury," *Spine*, Vol. 9, 1984, pp. 663–666.
[23] Penning, L., "Some Aspects of Plain Radiography of the Cervical Spine in Chronic Myelopathy," *Neurology*, Vol. 12, 1962, pp. 513–519.

Michael Kleinberger,[1] Rolf Eppinger,[2] Mark Haffner,[1] and Michael Beebe[3]

Enhancing Safety with an Improved Cervical Test Device

REFERENCE: Kleinberger, M., Eppinger, R., Haffner, M., and Beebe, M., **"Enhancing Safety with an Improved Cervical Test Device,"** *Safety in American Football, ASTM STP 1305*, Earl F. Hoerner, Ed., American Society for Testing and Materials, 1996, pp. 60–74.

ABSTRACT: The cervical spine serves two primary functions: (1) as a mechanical linkage that allows a large controlled range of head motions and (2) as a protective structure for the spinal cord that passes through the spinal canals of the vertebrae. Cervical injuries involving fracture or dislocation of the vertebrae often involve the spinal cord, leading to paralysis or even death. Although serious neck injuries have become relatively rare in American football since the adoption of new spearing rules and tackling procedures, the development of cervical protective equipment should further reduce both the severity and the frequency of neck injuries.

Many developers of cervical protective devices use anthropomorphic test devices, or ATDs, as physical surrogates for the athlete. Currently available ATDs are of limited biofidelity and ability to predict neck injuries under conditions involving head impact. This paper discusses the ongoing development of a new cervical test device with improved biofidelity in the frontal, lateral, and axial directions. A new transducer is proposed to measure dynamically the three-dimensional curvature along the length of the neck.

KEYWORDS: anthropometric test devices (ATDs), neck injury, cervical spine, injury criteria, finite element analysis

Introduction

The incidence of neck injuries in motor vehicle crashes totals in the hundreds of thousands every year. In 1993 alone, an estimated 340 000 cervical spine injuries occurred, which breaks down to approximately one injury every 1.5 min. If we consider only the more serious injuries (Abbreviated Injury Scale (AIS) $> = 3$), the occurrence drops down to around 9170 injuries; this is still orders of magnitude higher than the incidence of neck injuries in football. One factor that accounts for this difference is the number of participants in each activity. In 1993 there were over 175 million licensed drivers in 1993, compared with approximately 1.8 million participants in American football. Another factor is the higher energy levels associated with automotive crashes. Whether the injuries are sustained in the automotive or athletic environ-ments, the human neck remains the injured structure. For this reason, the large amount of

[1] Research engineers, Biomechanics Division, National Highway Traffic Safety Administration, NRD-12, 400 7th St., SW, Washington, DC 20590.
[2] Chief, Biomechanics Division, National Highway Traffic Safety Administration, NRD-12, 400 7th St., SW, Washington, DC 20590.
[3] Research engineer, Vehicle Research and Test Center, National Highway Traffic Safety Administration, East Liberty, OH 43319-0337.

research conducted for automotive or other types of crashes can be applied to the study of football injuries.

Athletic performance and typical human responses to various input conditions are routinely investigated using volunteers. Volunteer testing is limited, however, to noninjurious loading. To extend our knowledge into the realm of injury mechanisms and tolerances requires the use of a human surrogate. Surrogates can take many different forms, such as cadavers, animals, or a physical approximation to the human anatomic structure. This latter example includes the anthropomorphic test devices (ATDs or dummies) developed by the automotive and aeronautical research communities. The fact that these devices are durable, repeatable, and easily instrumented makes them a favorable choice for a surrogate.

Extreme care should be taken though when attempting to use these devices to evaluate injury potential under conditions for which they were not designed. An excellent example of this is the dummy neck being used in research to record neck loads during a head impact. The currently used Hybrid III dummy neck was designed to provide proper head rotation during a specified acceleration pulse applied to the base of the neck. This corresponds to a frontal crash in which the inertial loading from the head forces the neck into flexion without any head contact. The biofidelity of the dummy neck rapidly deteriorates once head impact occurs. This is largely due to the fact that the Hybrid III neck is too stiff when loaded in the axial direction compared with data from human cadaver tests. Another discrepancy between the Hybrid III and human necks is that the dummy neck does not allow any free rotation of the head relative to the neck. For these reasons, great care has to be taken when evaluating injury susceptibility based on experimental tests performed with currently available ATDs.

One solution to the problem is to design new ATDs which are more biofidelic in a wide variety of impact loading conditions. An exact replica of the human anatomic structure will probably never be created, but there is certainly room for improvement over current designs. The National Highway Traffic Safety Administration (NHTSA) is currently working on improvements to almost every component of the dummy anatomy. This paper will discuss the development of a new dummy neck with improved biofidelity in frontal flexion, lateral bending, and axial compression. Axial biofidelity is extremely important because serious cervical spine injuries often result from compressive loads directed through the cervical column.

Performance Specifications

The new cervical test device under development is primarily intended for use in frontal crash investigations. However, it is hoped that the same neck will be suitable for crash studies in all directions, including cases in which head impacts occur. A document entitled "Performance Criteria for a Biofidelic Dummy Neck" [1] was written to specify detailed requirements for neck biofidelity in all directions. This report attempts to compile all available neck response data to provide a set of criteria with which to judge a proposed dummy neck. In other words, if someone wishes to determine whether a given neck design is "biofidelic," its responses can be compared with the specifications in this document to judge its biofidelity. Kinematic and kinetic response corridors are provided for flexion-extension, lateral and oblique bending, axial compression-tension, and torsion.

Kinematic performance specifications are based largely on volunteer tests conducted at the Naval Biodynamics Laboratory (NBDL) by Ewing et al. [2–7] and analyzed by Wismans and Spenny et al. [8–13]. These data include translations and rotations of the head/neck complex during low velocity sled tests conducted in the frontal, lateral, and oblique directions. Plots are presented for neck angle (theta) and head angle (phi) versus time, as well as neck angle (theta) versus head angle (phi). Definitions of these angles are given in Fig. 1. Theta-phi plots indicate that the head rotation lags somewhat behind the neck rotation in a frontal crash.

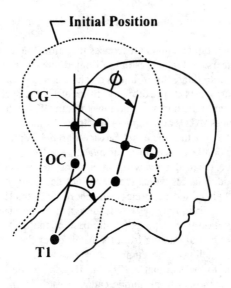

Initial Position

θ = Neck Angle
ϕ = Head Angle

FIG. 1—*Definition of head and neck angles.*

Initially, the neck flexes forward while the head remains horizontal. After approximately 30° of neck flexion, the head and neck rotate forward together.

Kinematic neck extension specifications consist of volunteer static range of motion tests [14–18] and dynamic volunteer tests conducted by the Japan Automobile Research Institute [19]. The dynamic data is very recent and is currently being analyzed for inclusion in the performance document.

Kinetic performance specifications consist primarily of torque versus angle corridors developed by Mertz et al., Patrick, and Chou [17,20–22]. Corridors are based on plots of the moment calculated at the occipital condyles (OC) versus head rotation with respect to the laboratory reference frame. These data are considered necessary, but not sufficient, for fully defining neck response, because they do not include translational requirements of the head relative to first thoracic vertebrae, T1. Additionally, these corridors cannot demonstrate response dependence on acceleration severity because they are developed without respect to time. The necessary time-dependent translational requirements have been incorporated into the performance specification document [1].

Human cadaver tests conducted by Yoganandan and Pintar [23–26] form the basis for the axial compressive specification. These researchers found the average compressive neck stiffness for a cadaveric specimen under quasistatic loading to be approximately 159 N/mm, with a standard deviation of 34 N/mm. The Hybrid III neck is approximately four to five times stiffer than the human cadaver. The 159-N/mm average value is considered a lower bound because the cadaveric specimens do not have any active musculature. Muscles serve to increase the stability of the neck, thereby stiffening the structure. The acceptable range of stiffness values is being taken as 159 to 227 N/mm that covers the mean plus two standard deviations.

Cadaver tests performed by Myers et al. [27] provide data for the torsional specifications. They suggest that a piecewise linear model with an initial load-free region, followed by a high stiffness region, adequately models the passive neck response to rotation. The initial load-free rotation was 66.8°, followed by a region with a mean torsional stiffness of 0.472 N-m/degree. Additionally, they reported that over half of the rotation occurs at the atlantoaxial joint.

Design Approach

Initial design attempts focused on a single deformable column with a hollow elliptical cross section. These initial designs were unsuccessful as a result of buckling of the hollow column during bending. The current design uses five deformable butyl rubber discs, separated by aluminum spacer plates. The cross sections of the rubber discs are elliptical with an interior circular hole that can be defined by three geometric parameters; namely, the A-P minor axis (b), the lateral major axis (a), and the radius of the circular hole (r). Figure 2 shows a schematic of the disc cross section.

Responses in all three primary directions (frontal flexion, axial compression, and lateral bending) can be optimized by varying the three geometric parameters. Flexion bending stiffness of the dummy neck is governed by the moment of inertia of the neck's cross section about an axis parallel to the lateral direction, given by $I_y = 0.25\pi (a^3b - r^4)$. Similarly, the neck's lateral bending stiffness is governed by the moment of inertia about an anterior-posterior axis, given by $I_x = 0.25\pi (ab^3 - r^4)$. Axial compressive stiffness is governed by the cross-sectional area, given by $A = \pi(ab - r^2)$, and the length of the compliant neck structure. The overall neck height was taken as 119 mm, the mean neck height of the NBDL volunteers. By entering the desired values for I_x, I_y, and A, the optimal values for a, b, and r can be calculated.

The design process began with the creation of a finite element model that satisfied the primary performance specifications; namely, frontal flexion, axial compression, and lateral bending. The current model, shown in Fig. 3, was created using the INGRID preprocessor along with the DYNA3D analysis program. It consists of approximately 3600 solid hexahedral elements, 100 shell elements, and 100 beam elements. The base plate, aluminum disc spacers, load cell blanks, and nodding blocks were modeled as solid rigid bodies. Solid elements were also used to define the deformable butyl rubber discs. The head was modeled as shell elements with additional discrete masses defined to provide proper inertial characteristics and location of the center gravity. Beam elements were used to define the three cables located anterior, posterior, and within the central canal of the neck. Contact between the cables and the aluminum plates were defined using a node-to-surface contact model.

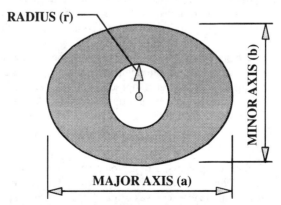

FIG. 2—*Cross section of butyl rubber discs.*

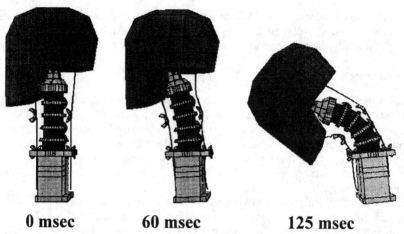

0 msec   60 msec   125 msec

FIG. 3—*Finite element simulation of prototype neck for frontal crash.*

The constitutive relationship of butyl rubber is a complex combination of phenomena, including hyperelasticity, strain rate sensitivity, and hysteresis. This complex behavior was simplified to a linear elastic material definition, with stiffness values obtained from dynamic coupon tests. The elastic modulus was originally estimated at 20 MPa.

Simulations were run for 8 and 15-g frontal flexion and also 7-g lateral bending. Acceleration curves and the corresponding velocity curves for each of these cases are shown in Fig. 4. These curves were obtained from the sled pulses used during the experimental testing of the prototype. Model results are shown in Fig. 5 through 7, respectively. Comparison of all response curves with the specified corridors was satisfactory. To keep the 8-g frontal flexion response within the corridor, it was necessary to have the 15-g response fall along the upper limit of the corridor. Axial compressive stiffness was calculated by hand, knowing the cross section and stiffness of the individual rubber discs.

Major differences between the new experimental design and the current Hybrid III are: (1) the inclusion of a low-friction pin joint at the occipital condyles to provide relatively free rotation and better agreement with NBDL volunteer kinematics and (2) a reduction in the cross-sectional area of the compliant sections to reduce the axial stiffness of the cervical column. Anterior and posterior spring-loaded cables have been included between the skull and thorax to obtain the proper lag response and to keep the head from rotating over the neck in the latter stages of the neck flexion. These cables also aid in setting the initial posture of the head/neck complex.

The torsional response reported by Myers et al. suggests the incorporation of a torsional joint in the dummy neck prototype to accommodate the relatively large amount of load-free rotation. However, since the frontal flexion response has been given the highest priority and, in most situations, relatively little torsion occurs in this crash mode, the torsional biofidelity of the neck will be addressed at a later time.

Prototype Fabrication and Testing

Based on the analytical design process, a first prototype neck was fabricated and tested on both a pendulum and sled. This prototype was unfortunately built from a different batch of 70-durometer butyl rubber than the one that was originally tested in the laboratory. The elastic modulus of this second batch was significantly less than the original batch, thus resulting in

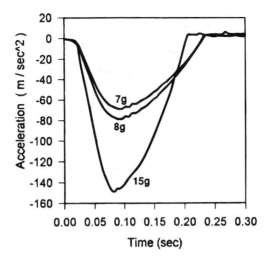

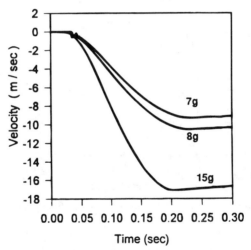

FIG. 4—*Acceleration and velocity curves used for experimental testing and analytical simulations.*

a prototype neck that was much too compliant. To account for this variability in material properties, a new set of dynamic coupon tests was conducted on the new batch. Revised values for the elastic modulus were inserted into the geometric optimization process to determine equivalent disc geometries for the new rubber material. Each butyl rubber disc had a height of 19.05 mm (0.75 in.), with geometric parameters as shown in Table 1. The upper three discs are identical, but the lower two discs were enlarged to distribute more evenly the stresses.

Kinematic results from frontal and lateral sled tests were analyzed and compared with the performance specification corridors. These results are shown in Figs. 8 through 10, along with plots of the Hybrid III responses. Although the responses do not lie within the specification

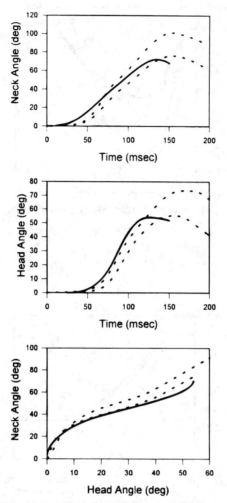

FIG. 5—*Simulation results for an 8-g frontal impact.*

corridors, they do show improvement over the Hybrid III neck. Axial stiffness for the neck structure is approximately 192 N/mm, which falls within the specified stiffness range. The axial stiffness of the Hybrid III is roughly 490 N/mm. Further work is required to satisfy the performance specifications for all three primary loading modes completely. The discrepancy between analytical and experimental responses is due primarily to the simplification in material characterization, made necessary by the unavailability of an accurate material model for butyl rubber within DYNA3D.

Instrumentation

Although generally accepted comprehensive neck injury criteria are not currently available, parameters expected to play an important role include the loads directed through the cervical column, the kinematics of the neck, and the position of the head relative to the neck. The

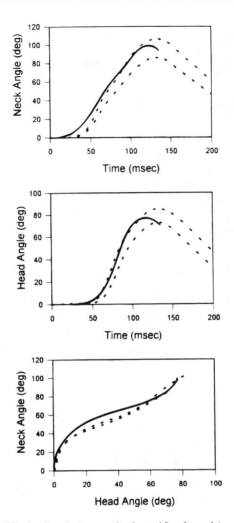

FIG. 6—*Simulation results for a 15-g frontal impact.*

importance of this latter parameter is evidenced by the difference in injuries observed between head-up and head-down contact in football.

Instrumentation in the new prototype dummy neck is intended to provide sufficient data for determining the necessary parameters for assessing injuries in frontal flexion, lateral bending, oblique bending, and axial compression. Head kinematics will be tracked using accelerometers and magnetohydrodynamic rotational velocity sensors. This instrumentation is currently available as an integral package within the Hybrid III head. Neck loads will be measured using a six-axis load cell both at the top and bottom of the cervical column. Additionally, loads carried through the cables and springs may be measured using button load cells. Figure 11 shows a design drawing of the prototype neck with the proposed instrumentation.

Measuring neck kinematics poses a more complex problem because the neck can bend in any direction, and may exhibit localized flexion and extension simultaneously. To measure the neck configuration dynamically, a new device called the Cervical Omnidirectional Bending

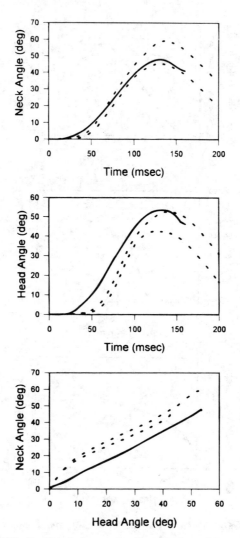

FIG. 7—*Simulation results for a 7-g lateral impact.*

TABLE 1—*Geometric design specifications for butyl rubber discs.*

Disc Number (1-sup., 5-inf.)	Major Semi-Axis, *a*, mm	Minor Semi-Axis, *b*, mm	Central Radius, *r*, mm
1, 2, and 3	31.2	23.5	6.35
4	34.4	25.9	6.35
5	37.6	28.4	12.3

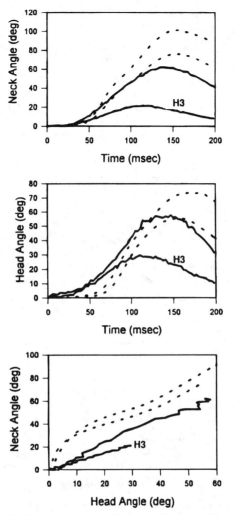

FIG. 8—*Experimental results for an 8-g frontal impact.*

Response Apparatus (COBRA) is under development. Mounted within the central canal of the neck, this device consists of thin plates instrumented with strain gages, mounted between discs, and arranged in alternating directions (AP and lateral). The device will dynamically record changes in curvature in each of the two directions. These responses can then be superimposed to obtain the three-dimensional shape of the neck. A prototype has been built, but has not yet been fully evaluated. A schematic diagram of the COBRA instrumentation is shown in Fig. 12.

Injury Assessment Strategies

Developing neck injury criteria promises to be a difficult task as a result of the complexity of the neck structure and the vast number of potential load paths through the cervical column. Dummy neck development is only one project within NHTSA's Neck Injury Research Program.

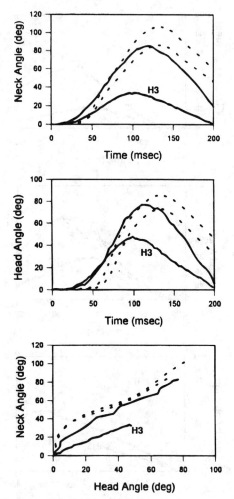

FIG. 9—*Experimental results for a 15-g frontal impact.*

This program is focused around the development of a highly detailed finite element model of the cervical spine [28]. Figure 13 shows a preliminary version of this model, including all vertebrae, discs, and ligaments. Musculature will be added to the model after it has been validated against cadaveric experimental data. Addition of musculature will enable the model to represent better a living human subject.

Data required for the development and validation of the analytical model are being provided by cadaver studies being conducted at two research institutions. These studies are investigating cervical injury mechanisms for both inertial and contact loading. Isolated tissue tests provide data for model development, whereas full cervical tests provide validation data. Failure tests provide valuable tolerance limits for the various structures in the neck that is essential for the development of neck injury criteria.

Once the model is validated, recorded results from dummy tests with a suitable prototype neck can be used to drive the analytical model. Loads or displacements or both measured in the dummy neck during a specific type of crash can be applied to the analytical model. It is

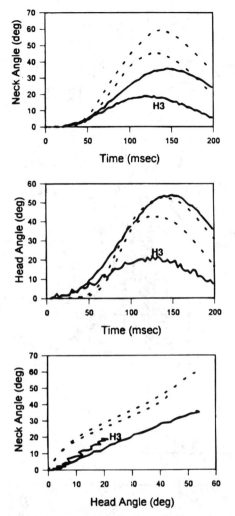

FIG. 10—*Experimental results for a 7-g lateral impact.*

anticipated that model results will then be useful to predict whether or not that particular loading condition would cause a cervical injury.

Future Design Efforts

The current prototype neck was designed as a stand-alone component and may not be completely compatible with the dummy torso. Spring housings in the current design to allow pretensioning of the cables will need to be redesigned to fit within the torso. The base of the neck needs to be attached to the torso so that the T1 level of the neck is positioned at the anatomically correct location. The T1 location in the neck is one segment superior to the base, making the most inferior spacer plate equivalent to the T1 position. Once a manufacturable design that is compatible with the full dummy is established, a final prototype will be molded and attention will turn to completing development of the instrumentation. COBRA development

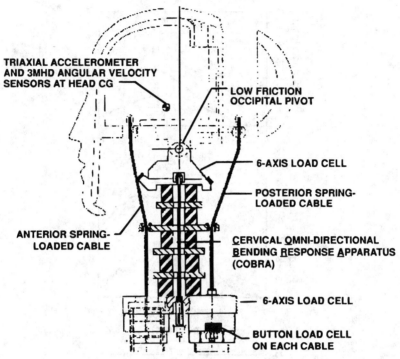

FIG. 11—*Design drawing of prototype dummy neck with proposed instrumentation.*

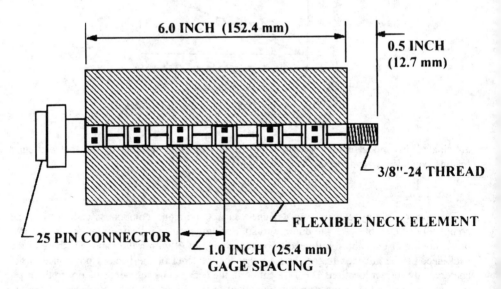

FIG. 12—*Schematic drawing of Cervical Omnidirectional Bending Response Apparatus (COBRA).*

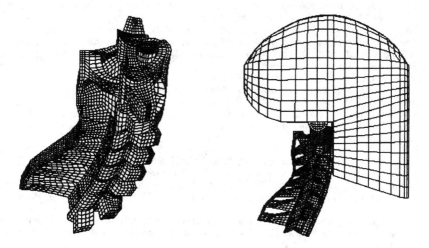

FIG. 13—*Finite element model of anatomic cervical spine.*

has already begun, and the first prototype will soon be tested to determine its feasibility. In addition, upper and lower neck load cells will be designed to fit within the geometric constraints of the new neck.

As was mentioned above, for most situations, relatively little neck torsion occurs during a frontal impact. However, in some "out of position" occupant impacts in airbag-equipped vehicles, it is possible for the airbag to contact the side of the face or chin or both of the dummy and cause torsional loading of the neck. For this configuration, as well as for side impacts, torsional biofidelity will be evaluated and, if found useful, incorporated into the next modification of the dummy neck prototype.

Acknowledgments

The authors would like to extend their thanks to Kathy Klinich at the Transportation Research Center in East Liberty, Ohio for her efforts in writing the performance document and analyzing test data from the pendulum and sled tests conducted on the dummy neck prototype.

References

[1] Klinich, K., Beebe, M., and Pritz, H., "Performance Criteria for a Biofidelic Neck," National Highway Traffic Safety Administration, Vehicle Research and Test Center Event Report, Aug. 1992.
[2] Ewing, C. L., Thomas, D. J., Beeler, G. W., Patrick, L. M., and Gillis, D. B., "Dynamic Response of the Head and Neck of the Living Human to -Gx Impact Acceleration," in *Twelfth Stapp Car Crash Conference Proceedings,* SAE Paper 680792, SAE, Warrendale, PA, 1968.
[3] Ewing C. L., Thomas, D. J., Patrick, L. M., Beeler, G. W., and Smith. M. J., "Living Human Dynamic Response to -Gx Impact Acceleration, Part II—Accelerations Measured on the Head and Neck," in *Thirteenth Stapp Car Crash Conference Proceedings,* SAE Paper 690817, SAE, Warrendale, PA, 1969.
[4] Ewing C. L. and Thomas, D. J., "Torque vs. Angular Displacement Response of Human Head to -Gx Impact Acceleration," in *Seventeenth Stapp Car Crash Conference Proceedings,* SAE Paper 730976, SAE, Warrendale, PA 1973.
[5] Ewing, C. L., Thomas, D. J., Lustick, L., Becker, E., Willems, G., and Muzzy, III, W. H., "The Effect of the Initial Position of the Head and Neck on the Dynamic Response of the Human Head

and Neck to -Gx Impact Acceleration," in *Nineteenth Stapp Car Crash Conference Proceedings*, SAE Paper 751157, SAE, Warrendale, PA, 1975.

[6] Ewing, C. L., Thomas, D. J., Lustick, L., Muzzy, III, W. H., Willems, G., and Majewski, P. L., "The Effect of Duration, Rate of Onset, and Peak Sled Acceleration on the Dynamic Response of the Human Head and Neck," in *Twentieth Stapp Car Crash Conference Proceedings*, SAE Paper 760800, SAE, Warrendale, PA, 1976.

[7] Ewing, C. L., Thomas, D. J., Majewski, P. L., Black, R., and Lustick, L., "Measurement of Head, T1, and Pelvis Response to -Gx Impact Acceleration," in *Twenty-first Stapp Car Crash Conference Proceedings*, SAE Paper 770927, SAE, Warrendale, PA, 1977.

[8] Wismans, J. and Spenny, C. H., "Performance Requirements for Mechanical Necks in Lateral Flexion," in *Twenty-seventh Stapp Car Crash Conference Proceedings*, SAE Paper 831613, SAE, New York, 1983.

[9] Wismans, J. and Spenny, C. H., "Head-Neck Response in Frontal Flexion," in *Twenty-eighth Stapp Car Crash Conference Proceedings*, SAE Paper 841666, SAE, Warrendale, PA, 1984.

[10] Wismans, J., "Preliminary Development Head-Neck Simulator" DOT-HS-807-034, Aug. 1986.

[11] Wismans J., van Oorschot, H., and Woltring, H. J., "Omni-Direction Human Head-Neck Response," in *Thirtieth Stapp Car Crash Conference Proceedings*, SAE Paper 861893, SAE, Warrendale, PA, 1986.

[12] Wismans, J., et al., "Comparison of Human Volunteer and Cadaver Head-Neck Response in Frontal Flexion," in *Thirty-first Stapp Car Crash Conference Proceedings*, SAE Paper 872194, SAE, Warrendale, PA, 1987.

[13] Spenny, C. H.,"Analysis of Head Response to Torso Acceleration," DOT-HS-807-159, DOT-TSC-NHTSA-86-5, Dec. 1987.

[14] Snyder, R. G., et al., "Bioengineering Study of Basic Physical Measurements Related to Susceptibility to Cervical Hyperextension-Hyperflexion Injury," University of Michigan Highway Safety Research Institute, UM-HSRI-BI-75-6, 1975.

[15] Glanville, A. D. and Kreezer, G., "The Maximum Amplitude and Velocity of Joint Movements in Normal Male Human Adults," *Human Biology*, 1937.

[16] Melvin, J. W., et al., "Advanced Anthropomorphic Test Device Development Program: Concept Definition," U.S. Department of Transportation, Sept. 1985.

[17] Patrick, L. M. and Chou, "Response of the Human Neck in Flexion, Extension, and Lateral Flexion," Vehicle Research Institute, VRI-7-3, SAE, Warrendale, PA, 1976.

[18] Schneider, L. W., et al., "Biomechanical Properties of the Human Neck in Lateral Flexion," in *Nineteenth Stapp Car Crash Conference Proceedings*, SAE Paper 751156, SAE, Warrendale, PA, 1975.

[19] Ono, K. and Kanno, M., "Influences of the Physical Parameters on the Risk to Neck Injuries in Low Impact Speed Rear-End Collisions," in *International IRCOBI Conference on the Biomechanics of Impacts*, BRON, France, 1993.

[20] Mertz, H. J., "The Kinematics and Kinetics of Whiplash" Ph.D. Dissertation, Wayne State University, Detroit, 1967.

[21] Mertz, H. J. and Patrick, L. M., "Strength and Response of the Human Neck," in *Fifteenth Stapp Car Crash Conference Proceedings*, SAE Paper, 710855, SAE, Warrendale, PA, 1971.

[22] Mertz, H. J., Neathery, R. F., and Culver, C. C., "Performance Requirements and Characteristics of Mechanical Necks," in *Human Impact Response: Measurement and Simulation*, W. F. King, and H. J., Mertz, Eds., Plenum Press, New York, 1973.

[23] Pintar, F. A., et al.,"Kinematic and Anatomical Analysis of the Human Cervical Spinal Column Under Axial Loading," in *Thirty-third Stapp Car Crash Conference Proceedings*, SAE Paper 892436, SAE, Warrendale, PA, 1989.

[24] Yoganandan, H., Sances, A., and Pintar, F. A., "Biomechanical Evaluation of the Axial Compressive Responses of the Human Cadaveric and Mannikin Necks," *Journal of Biomechanical Engineering*, 1989.

[25] Pintar, F. A., et al., "Biodynamics of the Total Human Cadaveric Cervical Spine," in *Thirty-fourth Stapp Car Crash Conference Proceedings*, SAE Paper 902309, SAE, Warrendale, PA, 1990.

[26] Yoganandan, N., et al., "Strength and Motion Analysis of the Human Head-Neck Complex," *Journal of Spinal Disorders*, Vol. 4, No. 1, 1991.

[27] Myers, B. S., et al., "Responses of the Human Cervical Spine to Torsion," in *Thirty-third Stapp Car Crash Conference Proceedings*, SAE Paper 892437, SAE, Warrendale, PA, 1989.

[28] Kleinberger, M., "Application of Finite Element Techniques to the Study of Cervical Spine Mechanics," in *Thirty-seventh Stapp Car Crash Conference Proceedings*, SAE Paper 933131, SAE, Warrendale, PA, 1993.

James C. Otis[1] and Albert H. Burstein[1]

A Proposed Method for Evaluating Neck Protection Equipment

REFERENCE: Otis J. C. and Burstein, A. H., **"A Proposed Method for Evaluating Neck Protection Equipment,"** *Safety in American Football, ASTM STP 1305*, Earl F. Hoerner, Ed., American Society for Testing and Materials, 1996, pp. 75–82.

ABSTRACT: The catastrophic nature of cervical spine injuries in football, although the incidence of these injuries is infrequent, has led to recent attempts to develop new methods of neck protection. Currently, no performance standards or test standards exist for neck protection equipment to assure the user that there would be a reduction in the risk of catastrophic neck injury. Additionally, no performance standards or test standards exist to assure that there would not be an increased risk of injury to other portions of the user's body or to the opponent's, and to assure that the equipment would perform adequately from a structural standpoint. Thus, a need arises to develop a standardized method for evaluating neck protection equipment. A proposed method for evaluating such equipment consisting of an analytical screening protocol and a physical test is presented.

KEYWORDS: neck protection, test standards, cervical spine

Introduction

The incidence of catastrophic neck injuries occurring during football games increased in the 1960s with the development of improved helmet-face mask protective systems. Although the helmet-face mask system reduced the number of head and facial injuries, it encouraged the use of the head as a primary contact point during blocking and tackling activities in football. As a result of the increased use of the head in activities such as spearing, the number of catastrophic neck injuries increased, as the cervical spine was subjected to more frequent and higher intensity loads [1]. The implementation of rule changes prohibiting the use of the helmet to butt or ram an opponent resulted in a reduction in catastrophic cervical spine injuries. Furthermore, better education of both coaches and players contributed to additional reductions in the frequency of catastrophic cervical spine injuries. Additionally, these injuries are seen during other sporting activities such as hockey and horse racing, where the number of injuries has not decreased. It is, therefore, the catastrophic nature of these infrequent injuries that has led to recent attempts to develop new methods of neck protection. Currently, no performance standards or test standards exist for neck protection equipment to provide any assurance to the user that there would be a reduction in the risk of catastrophic neck injury. Also, no performance standards or test standards exist to assure that there would not be an increased risk of injury to other portions of the user's body or to the opponent's, and to assure that the equipment would perform adequately from a structural standpoint. Thus, a need arises to

[1] Senior scientists, Department of Biomechanics and Biomaterials, The Hospital for Special Surgery, 535 E. 70th St., New York, NY 10021.

develop a standardized method for evaluating neck protection equipment. The method we propose consists of an analytical screening protocol and a physical test.

Analytical Screening

Two examples of neck protection systems which are in various stages of development are the air bag collar, which uses technology of the type used in the automotive industry, and the Protec system, a double helmet system which is designed to transmit impact loads away from the head and neck of the player, bypassing the shoulders, and distributing the forces over a wide area of the upper chest and upper back. Conceptually, these two systems are quite different, and it is evident that a spectrum of protection systems using different principles and technologies can be anticipated. As a result, a method of analytical screening is proposed that would: (1) determine whether a neck protection system meets basic, broadband requirements; (2) provide substantial cost savings by not requiring the development of a spectrum of physical tests to accommodate the potentially wide range of devices; and (3) permit the behavior of the neck protection system to be examined under simulated dynamic conditions. Thus, analytical screening would be beneficial for not only determining whether systems meet broadband requirements, but it would also provide a means of conducting analyses that would assist in the development of physical test systems.

Prior studies have been conducted which lend themselves to the development of an analytical screening protocol. An analytical model that uses the measured load versus deformation parameters for a helmet and the approximate load versus deformation parameters for the neck has been constructed to examine impact situations capable of generating loads that give rise to compression, buckling, and local hyperflexion failure [2]. The three-degree-of-freedom model assumes that the cervical spine is in an anatomically straight position, and it allows for the helmet wearer to impact or to be impacted by a moving mass. The model allows the helmet, head, cervical spine, and a portion of the trunk to move along a straight line coincident with the axis of the neck (Fig. 1). The load deflection characteristics of the neck are defined so that 4500 N of compressive force occurs with 23 mm of compression over the length of the cervical spine.

Results for a simulated impact are illustrated for a player impacting a fixed object at 4.6 m/s with an effective torso mass of 36 kg (Fig. 2). Typically, it is seen that the helmet force reaches a peak as the head begins to rebound. The displacement curve for the torso demonstrates that the torso continues to move at nearly a constant velocity throughout the simulated impact. The relative forward displacement of the torso as compared to the head results in compression of the cervical spine, as is evident from the rapid increase of the neck force, until the failure load of 4500 N is achieved. Figure 3 illustrates a comparison of five different helmets for the condition of an impact into a fixed barrier at 4.6 m/s with an effective torso mass of 36 kg. The model predicted catastrophic injuries regardless of the type of helmet; however, there were some temporal differences in performance with respect to occurrence of the failure load. The most rapid rate of load transfer to the neck occurred with the Shoei motorcycle helmet followed by the SK600 hockey helmet. Figure 4 illustrates the insensitivity of the generated neck force up to the failure load of 4500 N as the effective torso mass is varied from 36 to 9 kg. An understanding of the sensitivity of the system to variations in torso mass can be helpful in developing physical test systems for neck protection devices. In contrast, it can be seen in Fig. 5 that the rate at which force develops in the neck is quite sensitive to variations in impact velocity. Lastly, in Fig. 6, the rate of head deceleration for the different helmet systems clearly illustrates that, at the modest impact velocities encountered in football games, football helmets offer better impact protection for the head than do the motorcycle and hockey helmets, and that all helmets need to be designed to provide head protection at higher impact

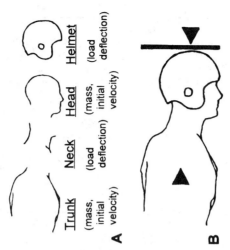

FIG. 1—(a) *The composite model consists of a trunk mass, a nonlinear spring cervical spine, a head mass, and a nonlinear spring-damped helmet load-deflection function. The basic law of dynamics (F = MA) characterizes the system. (b) The model, representing the axial loading injury condition, illustrates how the cervical spine is compressed between an abruptly decelerated head mass and the continued momentum of the body. (From Otis, J. C., Burstein, A. H., and Torg, J. S.;* "Mechanisms and Pathomechanics of Athletic Injuries," in Athletic Injuries to the Head, Neck, and Face, *J. S. Torg, Ed., Mosby Year Book, St. Louis, 1991, pp. 438–456. Used with permission.)*

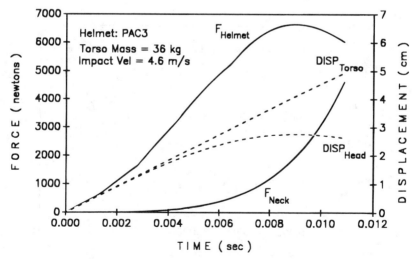

FIG. 2—*Force and displacement curves after impact with a fixed barrier demonstrates that the helmet force increased until a time at which the head rebounded (t = 8 ms). Torso displacement can be seen to continue at a nearly constant rate until the force limit was reached for the cervical spine. (From Otis, J. C., Burstein, A. H., and Torg, J. S., "Mechanisms and Pathomechanics of Athletic Injuries," in Athletic Injuries to the Head, Neck, and Face, J. S. Torg, Ed., Mosby Year Book, St. Louis, 1991, pp. 438–456. Used with permission.)*

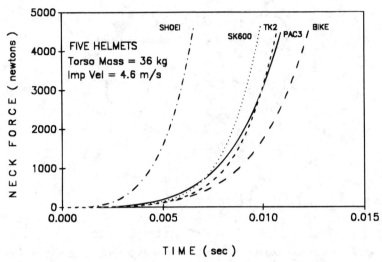

FIG. 3—*The neck force histories using five different helmets characterized in the simulation with an impact velocity of 4.6 m/s and a torso mass of 36 kg, demonstrating temporal differences in performance with respect to the onset of the failure load. (From Otis, J. C., Burstein, A. H. and Torg, J. S., "Mechanisms and Pathomechanics of Athletic Injuries,"* in Athletic Injuries to the Head, Neck, and Face, *J. S. Torg, Ed., Mosby Year Book, St. Louis, 1991, pp. 438–456. Used with permission.)*

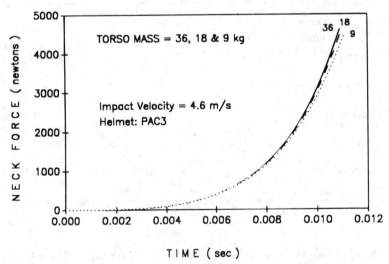

FIG. 4—*The neck histories for variations in torso mass from 36 to 9 kg with impact velocity remaining constant at 4.6 m/s (From Otis, J. C., Burstein, A. H., and Torg, J. S., "Mechanisms and Pathomechanics of Athletic Injuries,"* in Athletic Injuries to the Head, Neck, and Face, *J. S. Torg, Ed., Mosby Year Book, St. Louis, 1991, pp. 438–456. Used with permission.)*

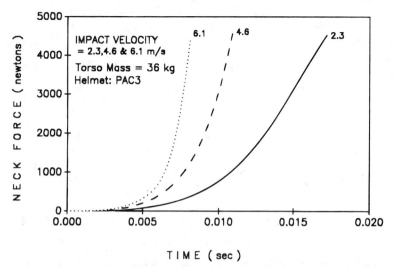

FIG. 5—*The neck force histories are illustrated for variations in impact velocity from 2.3 to 6.1 m/s with use of a constant torso mass of 36 kg. (From Otis, J. C., Burstein, A. H., and Torg, J. S., "Mechanisms and Pathomechanics of Athletic Injuries," in* Athletic Injuries to the Head, Neck, and Face, *J. S. Torg, Ed., Mosby Year Book, St. Louis, 1991, pp. 438–456. Used with permission.)*

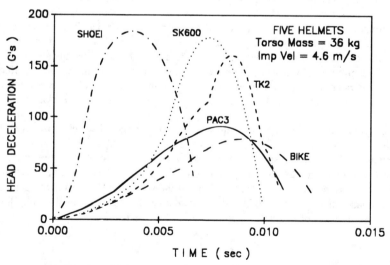

FIG. 6—*Simulated head decelerations associated with the five different helmets tested are illustrated with use of a constant torso mass and impacting velocity. (From Otis, J. C., Burstein, A. H., and Torg, J. S., "Mechanisms and Pathomechanics of Athletic Injuries," in* Athletic Injuries to the Head, Neck, and Face, *J. S. Torg, Ed., Mosby Year Book, St. Louis, 1991, pp. 438–456. Used with permission.)*

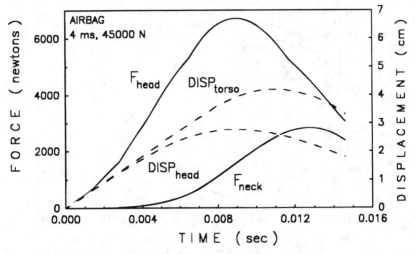

FIG. 7—*With a deployment delay time of 4 ms and the collar air bag force maintained at 45 000 N, the simulation produces no fractured cervical spine.*

velocities. Thus, even a simple analytical model can examine some aspect of the head protection offered by new devices which are intended to affect neck loading.

We examined the utility of analytical screening in determining the feasibility of using a collar air bag at the base of the helmet to transfer load to the shoulders, thus providing neck protection [3]. The model allowed parameters of bag deployment time and axial force generating capacity of the collar air bag to be investigated. It was determined that the combination of a 4-ms deployment time and a 45 000-N compressive force capability was necessary (Fig. 7) to incorporate a collar air bag into a cervical spine protection device. Thus, in the case of the air bag, analytical screening demonstrated that the available technology at that time would not permit successful use of a collar air bag. If the air bag becomes technically feasible, then it would be appropriate to investigate how deployment of a collar air bag would affect injury risk to the shoulder and upper torso region and, furthermore, it would be necessary to consider what injuries would be inflicted upon the player who is impacted by a tackler wearing such a device.

The analytical screening procedure relies heavily on the model which is based on an axial failure load. It is a first order approximation which considers the axial deflection mechanism, the mechanism that is responsible for the most catastrophic type of neck injury that occurs. In its present form, the model does not permit screening for more frequent, but less catastrophic, neck injuries. Furthermore, a prerequisite to using the screening protocol is the determination of the response characteristics of the neck protective device to be evaluated. This would necessitate some level of testing to identify these characteristics.

Injury Types

To date, the capability of the three-degree-of-freedom analytical model allows one to screen for injuries to the neck for a single mode, that of axial deflection. This mode was selected because it is the mechanism by which most catastrophic neck injuries occur. Clearly, any analytical screening procedure will need to consider those injury modes at the neck that are presently high risk and high severity and, also, those that have the potential for becoming high risk and high severity as a result of an intervention. Non-neck injuries that are important to screen for are those that occur to the brain and those that occur to the opponent.

An analytical model to be used for screening neck protection equipment systems must include in its specifications the mechanical characteristics for the neck, head mass, trunk mass, head stiffness, scalp stiffness, input parameters for the helmet or other neck protection device, the tolerance to injury for the body part of concern, and the conditions to simulate. Presently, parameters are specified for a passive neck model; however, current research into the role of active muscle forces in providing neck protection has the potential for the development of an active model [4]. The sources of material available for the development of an analytical model include the biomechanical literature which specifies to varying degrees the tolerance to injury of various body parts. In addition, the automotive safety literature includes specification of parameters associated with the development of anthropomorphic test dummies. A current source of material that examines the role of human cervical muscles under forced lateral bending is presently available as a recent Ph.D. thesis [4].

Physical Test

The development of a standard physical test to evaluate neck protection equipment should consist of an impact barrier, a test dummy, and a defined trajectory for the motion of the test dummy. The impact barrier would be very rigid so that energy absorption is kept at a minimum; for example, a stiffness of approximately 1×10^9 N/m would be appropriate. The barrier's surface should allow different coverings to provide controlled friction. This would be consistent with recent studies [5] which demonstrated that fixation of head position at impact influences the likelihood and mode of catastrophic injury to the neck. To assess impacts which are other than perpendicular to the barrier, it should have a vertical orientation at $90 \pm 45°$ to the testing axis.

The trajectory of the dummy would be horizontal at the time of impact, so that a pendulum mechanism would be acceptable for controlling the motion of the dummy. The impact velocity of the test dummy would range from 1.5 to 10 m/s. The axis of the dummy, trunk, neck, and head would be adjustable to $\pm 15°$ with respect to the trajectory. Specifications for the dummy head might include the 10th through 90th percentile mass for a male and an elastic scalp.

Specifications for the neck would include an axial compressive stiffness that was exponential and achieve 4500 N at 23 mm of axial deflection. Flexion extension stiffness and lateral bending stiffness could be used to model static muscle load and passive muscle to stretch. Specifications for the trunk would include a mass compatible to that of the corresponding head mass. The trunk would be designed to accept the shoulder pads, extension or flexion stop pads, and any other devices deemed appropriate.

Instrumentation for the barrier would include a three-axis, high-frequency load cell at the impact surface. An axial load capacity of 45 000 N and a shear load capacity of 9000 N would be appropriate. The head would include a triaxial accelerometer. The neck would include a six-axis load cell at the first thoracic level. An axial load capacity of 22 500 N, a shear load capacity of 9000 N, and moment capacities of 200 N-m would be adequate.

Validation of the physical testing scheme could include a comparison of the test results of dummy impact with no helmet with the results of the analytical model under the same conditions. These studies could be conducted using axial alignment of barrier, head, and torso at velocities of 1.5 to 10 m/s. When analytical models allow for off axis loading, testing will also be conducted at angles up to 10° off axis. Using a standard helmet, similar comparison of the test results with the analytical model results.

The development of standards for neck protection devices is important to the future development and distribution of such devices. Presently, potential developers of neck protection systems operate with no guidelines. Many of these individuals are unfamiliar with the mechanisms of neck injury and would welcome standard guidelines and specifications that their devices must meet. Potential manufacturers need some guidelines by which to judge the efficacy and injury risk of new devices. Devices that have met national standards are more appealing to manufacturers particularly from the standpoint of liability. In a similar manner, it is of ultimate importance to those distributing devices and selling them in the marketplace to have some reference by which these products may be judged with respect to efficacy of reducing the risk of injury. Lastly, those individuals involved with sports programs and the purchase of sporting equipment are not capable, in most cases, of making decisions with respect to the safety value of these devices for their athletes. They need the guidance that performance standards can provide.

Conclusion

In summary, it is imperative to agree upon some method for evaluating neck protection equipment. The proposed combined analytical and physical test methodology is not final by any means; however, it uses existing technology, provides a way to approximate known accident conditions, and looks at first order effects. Admittedly, test dummies are not perfect models of humans; however, they are improving and can provide capabilities for adjustment of axial neck stiffness, incorporation of simple instrumentation, and provisions for adjusting alignment.

References

[1]   Torg, J. S., "Anecdotal Observations," in *Athletic Injuries to the Head, Neck, and Face*, J. S. Torg, Ed., Mosby Year Book, St. Louis, 1991, pp. 3–14.
[2]   Otis, J. C., Burstein, A. H., and Torg, J. S., "Mechanisms and Pathomechanics of Athletic Injuries," in *Athletic Injuries to the Head, Neck, and Face*, J. S. Torg, Ed., Mosby Year Book, St. Louis, 1991, pp. 438–456.
[3]   Burstein, A. H. and Otis, J. C., "The Response of the Cervical Spine to Axial Loading: Feasibility for Intervention," in *Head and Neck Injuries in Sports, STP 1229*, E. F. Hoerner, Ed., American Society for Testing and Materials, West Conshohocken, PA, 1994, pp. 142–153.
[4]   Lu, W., "An Analytical Computer Model of the Human Cervical Spine Under Axial Compression and Lateral Bending," Ph.D. Thesis, University of Waterloo, Waterloo, Ontario, Canada, 1994.
[5]   Myers, B. S., McElhaney, J. H., Richardson, W. J., Best, T. M., and Nightingale, R. W., "The Effect of End Condition on Neck Injury Potential," in *Abstracts of ASTM International Symposium on Head and Neck Injuries in Sports*, Atlanta, 1993.

Tim McGuine[1] and Steve Nass[1]

Football Helmet Fitting Errors in Wisconsin High School Players

REFERENCE: McGuine, T. and Nass, S., "**Football Helmet Fitting Errors in Wisconsin High School Players**," *Safety in American Football, ASTM STP 1305,* Earl F. Hoerner, Ed., American Society for Testing and Materials, 1996, pp. 83–88.

ABSTRACT: The purpose of this study was to evaluate if football helmets were correctly fitted in high school football players from 34 randomly selected Wisconsin public high schools. Helmets were evaluated for correct fit by certified athletic trainers with the consent of the head coach. Helmet fit was assessed by examining seven specific criteria selected from standardized helmet fitting guidelines. The criteria selected for examination were as follows: (1) 1-in. (2.5-cm) clearance above the eyebrows, (2) 2-in. (2.5-cm) minimum clearance from nose to face mask, (3) chinstrap centered and tight, (4) jaw pads snug to face, (5) hear holes aligned and tight, (6) adequate coverage of the posterior cranium, and (7) minimal anterior/posterior movement with pressure. Each of the criterion was visually and manually inspected by the certified athletic trainers while the helmet was being worn by the football player. Other collected information included helmet brand, who fit the helmet, and year in school for the football player. In 1671 helmets 3403 fitting errors were observed for an overall fitting error rate (mean ± SD) of 2.04 ± 1.40, range 0 to 7. Of the helmets, 15.4% (n = 258) had no fitting errors, 23.5% (n = 392) had one or two fitting errors, 22.2% (n = 371) had 3 errors, and 15.4% (n = 258) had 4 or more errors. Bike helmets had the highest fitting error rate (2.34 ± 1.45) and highest percentage of helmets with 4 or more errors, 22.6% (n = 113), but Riddell® helmets had the lowest rate (1.84 ± 1.34) and the lowest percentage of helmets with 4 or more errors, 11.9% (n = 99). Freshman players had the highest fitting error rate (2.56 ± 1.44), while senior players had the lowest rate (1.80 ± 1.29). The most common error, 43.3% (n = 724) was inadequate or excessive clearance above the eyebrows. The least common error, 2.9% (n = 49), was adequate coverage of the posterior cranium. Although football helmets cannot prevent all head injuries in high school football, a correctly fitted helmet may decrease the likelihood of sustaining such an injury. Further study in this area is warranted.

KEYWORDS: helmet fit, athletic equipment, injuries, chinstrap

Introduction

High school football enjoys tremendous popularity in the United States. One unique aspect of football is the reliance on extensive protective equipment to prevent injuries. It could be argued that the most crucial piece of equipment is the football helmet. Since the 1950s, the football helmet has undergone extensive design changes to enhance its protective ability. These changes came about in an effort to reduce the number and severity of head injuries. A helmet that is properly designed, maintained, and fitted probably also reduces the likelihood of milder injuries such as concussions [1–4].

[1] The authors are certified athletic trainers providing high school outreach to high schools through the University of Wisconsin Hospital Sports Medicine Center, Madison, WI 53705.

Previous studies have focused on the incidence of head injuries by studying player position and activity at the moment the injury occurred [5,6]. Recently, Zemper showed the rate of concussions varied significantly between helmet brands and models [7]. In these studies, it was assumed that the helmets worn by the players were fitted properly by team personnel, despite the fact that a proper fit probably affects the protective ability of the helmet.

We were concerned that helmets worn by high school football players were not properly fitted, and that poorly fitted helmets offer less protection than properly fitted helmets. A pilot study of 422 high school players in ten high schools found that 47.8% wore helmets with multiple fitting errors [8]. Three factors were thought to be responsible for the high percentage of helmets with fitting errors: (1) the grade of the player, (2) the helmet brand, (3) and helmet fitting procedures use by the coach.

The purpose of this study was to document the incidence of helmet fitting errors in greater detail in Wisconsin high school football players. We wanted to examine three factors affecting proper helmet fit including the grade of the player, the helmet brand, and who fit the helmet for the player.

Methods

All helmet inspections were carried out by twelve certified athletic trainers certified by the National Athletic Trainers Associations (ATCs) who took part in an in-service to become familiar with data collection and inspection techniques to evaluate the appropriate helmet fitting criteria. Helmet-fitting criteria selected for evaluation in this study were obtained by reviewing several medical sources and material from the helmet manufacturers [9–12]. The seven criteria included: (1) 2.54-cm (1-in.) spacing above eyebrows, (2) 5.08-cm (2-in.) minimal clearance from the nose to the face mask, (3) chinstrap centered and taught, (4) jaw pads snug to the face, (5) ear holes aligned with the ears, (6) adequate coverage of the posterior cranium, (7) minimal shell movement anteriorly or posteriorly with exterior pressure. To help standardize the evaluations, three criteria 2.54-cm clearance above the eyebrows, 5.08-cm minimal space from the nose to the facemask, and jaw pads snug to the face were checked by using a laminated helmet fitting card developed for use in the study. Measurement of the spacing above the eyebrows was made with a tolerance of 0.65 cm ($^1/_4$ in.) The chinstrap was visually inspected for correct centering while tautness of each was examined by trying to place two fingers between the chinstrap and chin. The ear canal had to be visible through the helmet's ear holes to be considered in alignment. The coverage of the posterior cranium was considered to be adequate if the helmet covered the external occipital protuberance. Minimal anterior/posterior shell movement was determined by grasping the top of the helmet and applying anterior and posterior pressure. If this movement caused the skin of the forehead to wrinkle instead of simply sliding over the head, the helmet was considered to meet this criteria. Thirty-six public high schools in Wisconsin were randomly selected for the helmet evaluations. Athletic directors and head football coaches at each school were contacted by phone to make them aware of the study and obtain permission to conduct the helmet evaluations. Thirty-three schools agreed to proceed with the study, and arrangements were made to carry out the inspection at each school during the first 5 days of pre-season practices. Each of the seven criteria was visually and manually inspected by an ATC for each player present at the practice. Each criterion was graded as correct (+) or incorrect (−), with the athletes and coaches being aware of how to make the helmet meet all seven criteria. Other information recorded at the evaluation included: (1) who actually fitted the helmet for the athlete, (2) the grade level of the athlete, (3) and helmet brand.

Frequencies were tabulated for the total number of fitting errors and specific fitting errors. The average number of errors per helmet for each group were analyzed by one way ANOVA and if significant differences were detected, post hoc analysis with Fisher's protected least significant difference procedure was carried out to look at the values between the different groups.

Results

Three thousand four hundred three fitting errors were detected in 1671 helmets for an overall fitting error per helmet rate of 2.04 ± 1.40. The distribution (range = 0 to 4+) of total fitting errors for each helmet is summarized in (Fig. 1). Only 258 (15.4%) of the helmets had no fitting errors, while 392 (23.7%) had one error and 1021 (61.9%) had two or more errors. The frequency of specific fitting errors (Fig. 2) ranged from 49 (2.9%) for inadequate coverage of the posterior cranium to 724 (43.3%) for improper clearance above the eyebrows.

Table 1 illustrates the fitting errors per helmet rate (mean $\pm$ SD) for each grade level. Freshman ($n = 355$) had significantly higher ($p < 0.05$) fitting errors per helmet than all other classes. In addition, sophomores ($n = 501$) had significantly higher ($p < 0.05$) fitting errors per helmet than juniors ($n = 414$) and seniors ($n = 401$).

Fitting errors per helmet for three distinct helmet brands, Riddell® ($n = 826$), Max-Pro ($n = 501$), and Air ($n = 499$) are found in Table 2. Helmets manufactured under the old label Bike are included with those manufactured by its successor under the name Air. In the sample, Other included older helmet brands that were unable to be identified. Air helmets had a significantly higher fitting error per helmet rate as compared to Max-Pro and Riddell at the $p < 0.05$ level. Max-Pro were also noted to have a significantly higher ($p < 0.05$) fitting error per helmet rate than Riddell.

Table 3 summarizes the number of fitting errors according to who fit the helmet for the athlete. Coaches ($n = 1053$), included all coaching personnel on the school staff who fit the helmet. The category Players ($n = 419$), refers to all athletes who fit their own helmet with minimal intervention from the coaching staff. Helmets fit by Other ($n = 199$), included those fit by adult equipment managers and certified athletic trainers on staff at the school or provided to the school in an outreach program. The number of fitting errors per helmet for Other was significantly lower than the rate for "Coaches" and "Player" at the $p < 0.05$ level.

Discussion

Many helmets (61.9%), had multiple fitting errors despite the fact that helmet manufacturers include fitting instructions with each helmet. Manufacturers have also produced posters and videos detailing proper helmet-fitting procedures and make these readily available to school and team personnel. Yet many coaches participating in this study commented that their knowledge of helmet fitting was limited, and they welcomed any information that could be provided.

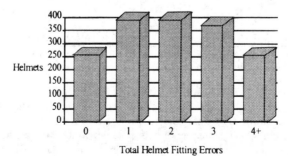

FIG. 1—*Distribution of total fitting errors in 1671 high school football players.*

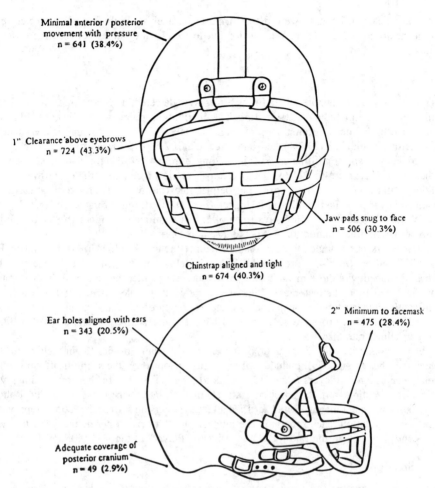

FIG. 2—*Frequency of specific fitting errors in 1671 high school football players.*

TABLE 1—*Helmet-fitting errors for each grade level.*

Parameters	Freshman	Sophomore	Junior	Senior	Total
Helmets	355	501	414	401	1671
Fitting errors	912	1017	752	722	3403
Errors per helmet	2.56 ± 1.44[a]	2.03 ± 1.37[b]	1.81 ± 1.36	1.80 ± 1.29	2.04 ± 1.40

[a]Freshmen had significantly higher ($p < 0.05$) number of errors per helmet than all other classes.
[b]Sophomores had a significantly higher ($p < 0.05$) number of errors per helmet than juniors and seniors.

Football helmets can offer an acceptable level of protection only if they are properly fitted and maintained. It could be argued that the criteria selected for determining proper helmet fit were too strict, producing a high number of helmet errors. Since there are no universal criteria for football helmet fitting, criteria were selected from the manufacturers' fitting instructions and published information in professional journals.

TABLE 2—*Helmet-fitting errors according to helmet brand.*

Parameters	Air	Max-Pro	Riddell	Other	Total
Helmets	499	501	826	5	1671
Fitting errors	1170	694	1525	14	3403
Errors per helmet	2.34 ± 1.45^a	2.03 ± 1.35^b	1.84 ± 1.34	2.89 ± 1.09	2.04 ± 1.40

[a]Air helmets had significantly higher errors per helmet ($p < 0.05$) than Max-Pro or Riddell.
[b]Max-Pro had significantly higher errors per helmet ($p < 0.05$) than Riddell.

TABLE 3—*Number of helmet-fitting errors according to who fit the helmet.*

Parameters	Coach	Players	Other	Total
Helmets	1053	419	199	1671
Fitting errors	2226	916	261	3403
Errors per helmet	2.11 ± 1.37	2.18 ± 1.42	1.31 ± 1.21^a	2.04 ± 1.40

[a]Helmets fit by other had significantly lower errors per helmet ($p < 0.05$) than helmets fit by coaches or players.

Surprisingly, 419 (25.1%) athletes in the sample were allowed to fit their own helmet. Coaches may be unaware of the risk of this potentially dangerous practice. However, in some cases, the high school players were as likely to fit their helmet as improperly as their coaches. This is supported by comparing the fitting error per helmet rates for "Coaches" and "Players," which are remarkably similar. This may indicate that coaches base their knowledge of what constitutes proper helmet fit by their previous experiences as players.

Lack of knowledge may have played a role in the frequency of some fitting errors. Numerous players were unaware of how their football helmet should fit and desired a level of comfort associated with a loose fit. Inflating air bladders to their proper levels helped eliminate excessive anterior/posterior movement; however, many athletes complained the helmet was now "too tight" when this error was corrected. Six hundred seventy-four (40.3%) players wore helmets with chinstraps that were not aligned or tight. Because of the decrease in comfort, many of the players were reluctant to correct the problem if they had a nonpadded chinstrap. It became clear that some players would adjust their helmet to make it less tight if they were given the chance. This points out the need for systematic helmet rechecks throughout the season.

Helmets with fitting errors could generally be divided into two groups. The first group included helmets with one or two errors (47.2%) that could often be corrected with minimal intervention. This intervention consisted of tightening the chinstrap, replacing small jaw pads with larger ones, or increasing the amount of air inflation, when possible, in the helmets. The second group was comprised of helmets with four or more errors (15.4%) that often indicated the helmet shell was too large and could not be made to fit, thus, requiring a replacement helmet that was smaller.

The high rate of helmet-fitting errors in freshman may be due to several factors. One likely cause may stem from the equipment distribution procedures used at many high schools. The high cost of helmets ($80 to $100) precludes many schools from having large numbers of helmets available to their athletes. Varsity players (usually juniors and seniors) are often given priority to select their equipment and will have the largest selection of helmets available to try on and fit. Subvarsity players (usually sophomores) are then allowed to draw their equipment and will have fewer helmets to select and fit. Freshmen are often the last grade to select their equipment, thereby greatly limiting their helmet choices and reducing the chance of having a helmet with a good fit.

A second reason for the high percentage of freshmen who had helmets with multiple fitting errors could be that the helmets are simply too large. Many coaches expressed frustration that even though they made their smallest players (usually freshmen) wear with the smallest helmets available the fit was not as good as with their other players. We estimated that between 5 and 15% of athletes had helmets that still fit poorly with maximum air inflation and extra large jaw pads.

Do each of the criteria play an equal role in the ability of the helmet to protect the athlete? Is there a combination of fitting errors that pose the greatest risk to the athlete? These questions are beyond the scope of this paper and could only be considered in a large scale epidemiological study of brain injuries in football players. Until such time as this is done, fitting criteria can only be selected based on the their perceived benefits to the protection afforded by the helmet.

Helmets would be easier to fit if the manufacturers worked with sports medicine professionals to provide a simple, easy-to-follow method for properly fitting football helmets. If large numbers of helmets cannot be made to fit using this method, a greater variety of helmet sizes should be provided so each helmet can be made to fit. In addition, we recommend that all football players be made aware of how their helmets should fit and how good fit enhances the protective ability of the helmet.

Conclusion

In this sample of high school football players, a large percentage wore helmets with multiple fitting errors. Furthermore, the number of fitting errors per helmet varied between the players grade in school, helmet brand, and who fit the helmet for the player. To increase football safety, coaches and players need to be educated in the crucial area of equipment fitting. Further studies that correlate specific fitting errors with an increased risk of concussion should be carried out.

References

[1] Cantu, R. C., "Guidelines for Return to Contact Sports After a Cerebral Concussion," *Physical Sports Medicine* Vol. 14, 1986, pp. 75–83.
[2] Gieck, J. and McCue, F. C., "Fitting of Protective Football Equipment," *American Journal of Sports Medicine* Vol. 8, 1980, pp. 192–196.
[3] Mueller, F. O., Blyth, C. S., and Cantu, R. C., "Catastrophic Spine Injuries in Football," *Physical Sports Medicine* Vol. 17, 1989, pp. 51–53.
[4] Storey, M. D. and Griffin, R., "Sub-dural Hematoma in a High School Football Player," *Physical Sports Medicine*, Vol. 11, 1983, pp. 61–71.
[5] Albright, J. P., McCauley, E., Martin, R. K., Crowley, E. T., and Foster, D. T., "Head and Neck Injuries in College Football: an Eight Year Analysis," *American Journal of Sports Medicine,* Vol. 13, 1985, pp. 147–152.
[6] Buckley, W. E., "Concussions in College Football: a Multi Variate Analysis," *American Journal of Sports Medicine,* Vol. 16, 1988, pp. 51–56.
[7] Zemper, E. D., "Analysis of Cerebral Concussion Frequency with the Most Commonly Used Models of Football Helmets," *JNATA* Vol. 29, 1994, pp. 44–50.
[8] McGuine, T. A. and Nass, S. J., "Evaluation of Football Helmet Fit in High School Football Players," *Medicine and Science in Sports and Exercise,* Vol. 26, 1994, p. S 13.
[9] Arnheim, D. D., *"Essentials of Athletic Training,"* 2nd ed., Mosby Year Book, St. Louis, 1991, pp. 102–104.
[10] "How to Properly Fit the Air Helmet Systems," Athletic Helmet, Inc., Knoxville, TN, 1991.
[11] NCAA Committee on Competitive Safeguards and Medical Aspects of Sports, "Guidelines for Helmet Fitting and Removal in Athletics," *1991 NCAA Sports Medicine Handbook,* M. Benson, Ed., NCAA Sports Science, Overland Park, KS, 1991, pp. 51–52.
[12] "Riddell Helmet Care and Fitting Instructions," Riddell, Inc., Chicago, 1991.

C. A. "Dewey" Morehouse[1]

The Process of Certification of Protective Equipment for Sports

REFERENCE: Morehouse, C. A., "**The Process of Certification of Protective Equipment for Sports**," *Safety in American Football, ASTM STP 1305,* Earl F. Hoerner. Ed., American Society for Testing and Materials, 1996, pp. 89–93.

ABSTRACT: The details of the three essential phases for the certification of protective equipment for sports in the United States are described in this paper. The initial phase includes the necessary prerequisites for the development of written objective, scientific standards based on physical tests consistent with current engineering technology. The recommended features of a certification council including the employment of a third party validator for the adherence of products to available standards are outlined in the second phase. The third and final phase consists of the communication and cooperation of rules-making organizations necessary for proper compliance and the ultimate safety of the sports participants. The model used for illustrating the entire process of certification is the Hockey Equipment Certification Council (HECC), a volunteer organization established in 1976 for the certification of ice hockey equipment. The fact that mandated use of certified eye and face protection has reduced the eye and facial injuries in organized ice hockey by over 99% since the program was initiated in 1978 is evidence that certification can be very effective in the reduction of injuries if properly organized and administered.

KEYWORDS: standards, certification councils, compliance, safety, injuries, athletic equipment, technology

The process of certifying protective equipment for sports consists of three basic components: (1) the development of standards, (2) the certification program or council, and (3) compliance and education. To use a familiar cliche, these three aspects are like the links of a chain, and the results of the certification process will only be as good as the weakest link. Also, to be most effective, the three parts must be linked together by effective communication. Some of the important characteristics of each phase will be discussed in this article, with an emphasis on the certification program.

The Development of Standards

ASTM's rules and regulations for the development of standards are well known. No attempt will be made to relate all their procedures in detail, but, certain essential elements of a viable standard will be emphasized.

First, a standard must be written in clear, concise, and coherent language. The true test to determine if this is achieved is if the standard can be accurately interpreted by a third party that was not involved in the writing of the document. The input during the process of developing the standard should come from three groups: consumers or users, producers, and general interest. This is what ASTM calls balanced representation. If the process is dominated by

[1] Professor Emeritus, Penn State University, 621 Old Farm Lane, State College, PA 16803.

consumers, it is possible that the standard will be so stringent that it may be impractical from manufacturing and economical standpoints. On the other hand, if the producer group dominates, the standard may not be stringent enough for adequate protection of the athletes. The general interest group, which includes researchers from universities, representatives of testing laboratories, and medical personnel, provides an expertise which neither of the first two groups possess. Normally, the actual wording of standards becomes a compromise among these three groups of individuals.

The standard should, when feasible, include objective physical tests often referred to as engineering tests that are described in detail and can be conducted in any testing laboratory given the correct equipment. The testing equipment should not be overly expensive and should be available commercially. If at all possible, common laboratory equipment should be used. When the equipment is specially built, engineering plans should be attainable, preferably in the Appendix of the standard.

The test methods must be both repeatable and reproducible. Repeatability means that a given laboratory generates consistent results. This is often called "within laboratory reliability." Reproducibility, on the other hand, refers to consistency of results among three or more laboratories or "between laboratory reliability." Both of these qualities are assessed by round robin tests involving a group of laboratories. Round robin tests also provide an estimate of the variability of test results. ASTM refers to this as a measure of test precision. If standard specifications for an item of protective equipment are prescribed based on a standard test method, test precision data provide an objective means for selecting a value for minimum performance with a higher probability for protection against injuries.

In addition, a test method must include a pretest calibration procedure and if electronic equipment is used, a posttest calibration should be specified. These calibrations make it possible to determine if the equipment is operating properly at the beginning of a testing session, and to detect electronic drift which sometimes occurs during a testing session.

Most individuals closely associated with football are aware that the National Operating Committee on Standards for Athletic Equipment (NOCSAE) has written a standard for the impact attenuation of football helmets. What many people do not realize is that this group does not certify football helmets as a result of a number of reasons, one of which is that the standard calls for a test procedure that is repeatable but not reproducible. In addition, the standard does not include a pretest calibration procedure, although it does include a posttest calibration to account for electronic drift. Because of these weaknesses in the standard, NOCSAE has resorted to a self-certification program. In this writer's opinion, the effectiveness of a self-certification program is questionable. This viewpoint is based on the number of head concussions that are currently being reported as occurring in our high school, college, and professional games. Assuming commercial companies are not cutting corners, the number of reported head concussions indicate that the standard should be more stringent. This could be accomplished readily by increasing the impact energy of the helmet drop test or lowering the Gadd Severity Index from its current maximum value of 1500 to 1200 or even to 1000. Such modifications in the standard would provide greater protection against concussions.

The Certification Program

After a suitable standard has been published, the second step in the certification process is to set up a certification program. Some organization or certification council such as the Hockey Equipment Certification Council (HECC) is needed to monitor continuously such a program. (Established in 1976, HECC is an independent volunteer organization consisting of consumers, manufacturers, and general interest personnel. Membership is open to all individuals interested in the improvement of the safety and play of all aspects of ice hockey.[2] An organization for certification should be nonprofit, independent of the standards-writing body, and be governed by a constitution that sets forth written guidelines for its operation. The essential elements of a constitution should include: (1) a statement of purpose; (2) the officers, their responsibilities, how they are elected, and the length of their terms; (3) who is eligible for membership; (4) requirements of meeting announcements and frequency of meetings; (5) finances and dues; and (6) standing committee structure.

The most important standing committee is a Certification Committee. This group should be representative of the membership and be balanced with equal numbers of producers, consumers, and general interest members. The preferable size of such a committee is at least six, but no more than ten members. If the group is too large, it is hard to find a meeting time that is suitable for all members, and it is very difficult to make timely decisions in large groups. There are difficult decisions that must be made continually. HECC's Certification Committee meets at least twice each calendar year, and often three or four times a year for all day meetings to conduct its business. There are always differences of opinions in the interpretation even of well-written standards and these are usually differences between a manufacturer's interpretation and the interpretation of the official validator. These must be heard and mediated by the Certification Committee.

The Certification Council should have an agreement in the form of a written contract with an independent testing laboratory stating the conduct and administration of the validation program. This independent body must have adequate equipment and technical personnel to conduct all tests required by the written standard or standards. It must not be controlled or operated by a producer, supplier, or buyer of a certified product. It should be a recognized testing laboratory with appropriate supervisory personnel to properly administer the program. The American National Standards Institute (ANSI) has a standard, Z34.1, entitled American National Standard Certification—Third Party Certification Program,[3] that stipulates in great detail the essential characteristics of third party validation. In the case of ice hockey, HECC has a contract with ETL/Inchcape Laboratories of Cortland, NY, part of an international corporation with testing laboratories in several countries.

ETL administers the entire certification program. As HECC's validator, they correspond with current and prospective manufacturers that subscribe to the various certification programs. Any and all manufacturers, upon request, are encouraged to join a specific program. Upon receiving such a request, they are sent a Procedural Guide which explains in detail how the program operates, including, but not limited to, the number of samples to be submitted, time intervals between tests, testing fees, and appeal procedures in case of a serious disagreement between the validator and the program subscriber. If the manufacturer agrees with these conditions and decides to subscribe to the program, a license agreement is signed that stipulates the obligations of the manufacturer as well as the consequences for program violations. The most serious consequence is decertification of a product or exclusion from the entire program.

Upon receipt of the signed License Agreement and the necessary samples, ETL conducts the tests according to HECC's adopted standards. If the product satisfies the requirements of the standard, the manufacturer is notified, and the estimated number of certification labels needed for the next three-month period are purchased.

In addition to performing initial tests, ETL conducts annual tests to continue the certification. Extra tests are necessary if a model change is made involving a difference in either construction

---

[2] Detailed information concerning its certification programs and membership applications are available from HECC Treasurer, Dr. Carl J. Abraham, Ph.D., 167 Willis Ave., Mineola, NY 11501, Tel. (516) 747-8400.

[3] American National Standards Institute, Inc., 1430 Broadway, New York, NY 10018.

or materials. All certified equipment is listed by make, model number, size, and date of last certification test. HECC distributes this list to all its members three or four times a year.

ETL/Inchcape personnel also make an annual visit to each manufacturer's plant or warehouse to inspect its production records, and to verify the quality control within the manufacturing process. Records of units sold in the United States must correspond to the number of certification labels purchased during the time interval between visits. A portion of the income from the sale of certification labels goes to HECC and is used for other aspects of the total program.

These labels have a special code for each manufacturer, so if uncertified hockey equipment appears at a retailer's establishment with a label on it, the manufacturer can be identified and warned that such breaches of contract are cause for decertification and exclusion from all HECC programs. No certified products can be sold in the United States unless they have a HECC sticker attached. These stickers are made so that they cannot be removed without destroying them. Stick-on labels are used in all programs instead of using embossments in the dies, because most manufacturers of ice hockey equipment are based in Canada and they sell products in both countries.

When a dispute arises between the validator and a manufacturer with regard to a test result or an interpretation of a standard which cannot be readily resolved, a written complaint is sent to the HECC Certification Committee by the manufacturer and a written statement of ETL's position is provided. It is then the task of this Committee to resolve this problem. Such situations arise continually, so the Certification Committee members are very active.

Another important standing committee of HECC is the Statistics and Research Committee. Its responsibility is to gather injury reports from any and all sources available in an effort to determine if the certified equipment being used in the field is actually preventing most of the injuries. These data may give some indication of the need for a more stringent standard, in which case the ASTM Subcommittee on Ice Hockey is petitioned to modify the appropriate standard. In the case of half shields or visors, the Canadian Standards Association (CSA) is contacted because ASTM does not have a written standard for these products, therefore, the CSA standard has been adopted by HECC.

Compliance

The third and final stage of the certification process is compliance. This involves the cooperation of the rules-making organizations for the sport. In the case of ice hockey, USA Hockey, the National Collegiate Athletic Association (NCAA), and the National Federation of State High School Associations (NFSHA) have all required that certified helmets and full-face protectors be worn in all sanctioned games. On the other hand, HECC has a certification program for skate blades in place, but none of the hockey rules-making bodies has felt it important enough to require that certified skate blades be worn in sanctioned competition. USA Hockey, however, does recommend that certified skate blades be worn. This is the current situation even though a number of serious injuries have occurred as a result of broken skate blades. Consequently, none of the companies manufacturing skate blades feels the necessity to join the certification program. This is mentioned only to emphasize the point that, unless rules-making bodies mandate the use of certified equipment, companies ordinarily will not voluntarily subscribe to a program because it does involve a financial outlay.

A certification council must assume the major responsibility of making the entire process function. Lists of certified equipment must be updated every few months, and these lists must be distributed not only to the athletic organizations, but also to the registered officials, for the purpose of monitoring players to determine if certified equipment is being worn at all times. Coaches and equipment managers need to be sent lists so that schools purchase only the models of equipment that are on the current certified lists. Retailers need to know what equipment to buy from wholesale representatives. In most cases of younger participants in nonschool programs, the parents must also be aware that only certified equipment can be worn in games. Additionally, it is valuable for these various groups to inform the certification council when certified protective equipment is not doing an adequate job of preventing injuries so that the standards-writing group can be petitioned to modify a standard accordingly.

In essence, open and effective communication is necessary between all three aspects of the certification process. It certainly should be recommended that the football community seriously consider formulating a plan for certification of its protective equipment. This recommendation is based on the large number of serious injuries, especially concussions, that are occurring in this violent contact sport, or as former Michigan State Football Coach, Duffy Daugherty, once termed it, *collision sport.*

A complete certification program with third party testing and mandated rules for use of equipment provides concrete benefits for players, parents, coaches, and producers. With certification, players have fewer injuries and can avoid a great deal of pain, suffering, and loss of playing time, thereby deriving greater enjoyment from participation. Parents are informed of what products to purchase with assurance that the products satisfy minimum standards for safety. Consequently, parents are relieved of some of the worries regarding serious injuries to their children. If parents are responsible for health care, they may save on insurance premiums. Coaches will also benefit from knowing which products to recommend for purchase, and from having healthier players a greater percentage of the time. They should also feel better knowing that their players are well protected. In addition, smaller budgets will be required for medical care. Manufacturers will experience fewer litigations, and when a litigation does occur, they will have a more effective defense. Thus, manufacturers will save on their liability premiums. Finally, all members of these groups should feel reassured that the game is being made as safe and enjoyable as possible for participants at all levels of play.

Management: Facilities

A. H. Mittelstaedt[1]

Football Fields and Facilities: Safety Guideline Concerns

REFERENCE: Mittelstaedt, A. H., "**Football Fields and Facilities: Safety Guideline Concerns,**" *Safety in American Football, ASTM STP 1305,* Earl F. Hoerner, Ed., American Society for Testing and Materials, 1996, pp. 97–99.

ABSTRACT: Football fields, known to most people as the pro/college stadium or the local field at the park or school grounds, are used at many levels of proficiency by players of all ages. Little attention is given to the differences imposed by variations in skill, size, training, equipment, and other human factors. Studies are being undertaken by the National and American Football Leagues, universities, the medical profession, and Players Association, as well as the National Federation of State High School Athletics Association, the National Athletic Trainers Association, and others. These organizations are studying factors such as physical conditioning, developmental and physical characteristics of players, types of training and scrimmaging, types of plays, defensive and offensive motions, blocks, tackles, interceptions, other techniques, protective devices, and other aspects of the game. There is no question that there is a cause-and-effect relationship between the players' performance, equipment, the facilities, and the injuries. It must be acknowledged that regardless of the surface, facility, or equipment, football has inherent risks. This paper addresses those aspects of the football field surface and other appurtenances that may be the cause of injury.

KEYWORDS: safety guidelines, football fields, surfaces, space, dimensions, injuries, prevention, play, control, administration

Football Fields and Facilities: Safety Guidelines

Football fields are known to most people as the local field at the park or school grounds. Unfortunately, the pro/college game is emulated by all others. The Pee Wee team and its adults organize and play as though they were televised; the junior or senior high school teams play as though they were being scouted, and adult clubs or pickup teams play for the money. However, little attention has been focused on the different situations created in these games because of variations in skill, size, training, equipment, and other human factors at the facilities.

Studies are being undertaken by the National and American Football Leagues, universities, the medical profession, the Players Association, as well as the National Federation of High School Athletics Association, National Athletic Trainers Association, and others as to conditioning, developmental size, and strength characteristics of the players, types of training and scrimmaging, types of plays, defensive and offensive motions, blocks, tackles, interceptions and other techniques, evasive and protective devices, and other aspects of the game. Some of these organizations are starting to undertake reviews of facilities, surfaces, equipment, shoes, padding, and helmets. Other professions are starting to examine injuries and resulting disabilities, and life expectancies of players through, for example, the National High School Registry, the National Institute of Occupational Safety and Health, and universities such as Ball State

[1]Executive director, Recreation Safety Institute, 39 Shadyside, Port Washington, NY 11050.

University in Indiana and the University of Iowa. There is no question that there is a causal relationship between a player's performance, equipment, the facility, and injuries. It must be acknowledged that regardless of surface, facility, or equipment, football has inherent risks.

This paper addresses those aspects of the football field surface and other appurtenances that can be the cause of injury. Unfortunately, a football field is usually related or referred to as either the professional stadium fields seen on television or the multiuse fields that are viewed at high schools. The football field is typically part of or enclosed by another sports facility, such as the quarter-mile running track, steeplechase, shot put, hammer and discus, high jump, pole vault, and broad jump. The field may also encompass soccer, lacrosse, or other field sports activities. The latter types of fields are necessary because of the lack of space, safety, and costs of preparing other level natural or synthetic turf spaces. The incorporation of these other functions often results in a compromise in safety and can provide conflicts with the participants of other sports with the potential to create hazardous situations.

The former type of perfected stadium or bowl for pro/collegiate sports far exceeds the pocketbook of most owner/operators, satisfying the demand for multiage group teams that wish to play football. The result is football fields that are designed for the sports-specific event or activity of football. If designed and constructed as an independently or singularly used facility, the following considerations must be addressed to reduce the number of injuries incurred during scrimmage, practice, or competition. The chapter "Safety Recommendations in the Design of Athletic and Sports Fields," in the book titled "*Natural and Artificial Playing Fields: Characteristics and Safety Features,*" published by the American Society for Testing and Materials, contains a section devoted to football fields and provides a basis for safety criteria. In addition to these components, the field, sidelines, end zone and surrounding area, and associated appurtenances should receive attention in the establishment of a football field.

Space

The area or dimension required for a football field should be reflective of the age and skill of the players involved. Six-man, eight-man, touch, and midget football require different sizes of playing fields. As a result, the survey monuments for pylon, line placement, and other fixtures must not interfere with the game. Synthetic treatment and types of lines are all affected by the space allocated to the level of use.

Surface

The surface is the most controversial aspect of the playing field. Literally, hundreds of commentators, coaches, and players have all set forth their views on the value of the different types of surfaces, but the jury is still out in that regard. There is no doubt that many factors are used in the selection of the surface, either synthetic or natural, and the type of surface performance. For example, when considering surface performance, the following preferences must also be weighed:

Play Preferences—These have been dominant in the discussion of surface selection. Concerns over traction, cushioning or softness, resilience, stopping or holding capability, turning or twisting giveability, starting, sliding, and impact attenuation are among the attributes being debated.

Owner Preference—A number of factors influence owners' selection preferences: construction costs, i.e., manufacturer's price, shipping charges, and installation fees; operation costs associated with color, glare, or reflection intensity and lining requirements; maintenance costs, i.e., cleaning and repair charges, fast drying, vacuuming, and line replacement costs; and longevity, i.e., discoloration, degradation, durability, repair work, logo use, and adaptability for other uses and traffic intensity.

In addition, many sports planners have personal perceptions of what may be the best type of surface, material or other factors to choose from. This list is by no means complete and other factors determine how a surface, whether natural or synthetic, may be judged. However, the time has come for these other factors to be discussed, evaluated, and tested in an impartial manner. Testing must also be expanded to include the types of shoes worn by players in relation to surface types.

Boxes or Viewing Area—The space for official or press personnel can vary, depending upon the type of field. Press personnel, including those from newspaper, radio, television, cable, or movies, should be cautioned against assuming positions that can interfere with the players. This is particularly important for photographers and television crews. Public personnel, including announcers and other speakers, should be alerted to placement of their equipment so that they do not interfere with the game. Spotters and game personnel, including coaching personnel and those under contract to record the game by audio/video or movies, should not have their tables and equipment placed so that they might interfere with the game. Scouts and other personnel, including those from the sanctioning body or other teams, can also interfere with the safety of those playing the game. Those individuals, if not in or about the grandstands, should be away from the play zone so as not to injure or be injured by the players.

Scoreboard—The type of scoreboard used will also be a result of the type of field and level of play. Scoreboards, particularly portable scoreboards, should be well out of the potential area of play. All cables, wires, controls, and other fastenings should be placed in locations or within barriers so as not to interfere with play.

Goal Posts—The type of goal posts used is critical to reducing injuries during collisions. They must have adequate padding to protect the player.

Lighting and Light Poles—The lighting and placement of lights are essential to provide proper lighting and complete illumination. Poles and stanchions should be well out of the way of play. Such elements of the football field require more attention to reduce injuries at every level of competition.

The concerns addressed in this paper must be finalized into definitive criteria to make football fields safer for all involved in the sport. This paper has opened the dialogue that must take place through established safety organizations such as the National Safety Council's public recreation committee or the Recreation Safety Institute.

Management: Surfaces

Richard D. Breland[1]

Standard Test Methods and Performance Standards for Synthetic Turf Playing Surfaces and Materials

REFERENCE: Breland, R. D., **"Standard Test Methods and Performance Standards for Synthetic Turf Playing Surfaces and Materials,"** *Safety in American Football, ASTM STP 1305*, Earl F. Hoerner, Ed., American Society for Testing and Materials, 1996, pp. 103–113.

ABSTRACT: Synthetic turf playing surfaces have been in use for over 25 years. A set of standard test methods and performance standards have evolved and are in widespread use to characterize synthetic playing surfaces and materials. A standard guide is being published that establishes a recommended list of test methods to be used for characterization of physical properties and comparison of performance properties of synthetic turf components and systems for athletic or recreational use.

A set of ASTM testing methods and various technical properties are described in compiling a complete synthetic turf system. Some values for required performance levels and typical measured values for synthetic turf components and systems are described. The typical values are subject to normal variation both in production control and in testing, especially when different testing laboratories or testing methods are involved.

Laboratory testing conditions are controlled at 65 ± 2% relative humidity and 21 ± 1°C (70 ± 2°F) unless otherwise noted in the standard test method. Testing in laboratories under markedly different conditions and techniques will give different test results in most cases.

The objective of this paper is to present Standard Test Methods and Performance Standards adopted for physical property characterizion of synthetic turf system components, artificial turf and synthetic turf systems.

KEYWORDS: synthetic turf, artificial turf, football surface, performance standards, test methods, playing surface, pile wear, tuft bind, compression resistance, grab tear, flammability, shock absorbancy, shoe traction, water permeability, relative abrasiveness, turf system

Introduction

Synthetic turf football and baseball playing surfaces have been in use for over 28 years. Testing programs, test methods, and performance standards have evolved and are used to characterize synthetic and natural turf systems.

Morehouse [1] reported that to achieve greater uniformity among surfaces and insure adequate durability, testing programs and scientific standards should be developed. To this end, ASTM Committee F-08 on Sports Equipment and Facilities has published ASTM Test Methods for Comprehensive Characterization of Synthetic Turf Playing Surfaces and Materials (F 1551) (Table 1). These tests methods and some values for required performance levels as well as typical measured values for synthetic turf components and systems are described.

[1] Breland Consultant and Service Company, P.O. Box 1403, Dalton, GA 30722-1403.

TABLE 1—*Performance test methods for synthetic turf surfaces.*

ASTM Test	Suffix	
		PILE FIBER
D 789		Melting point
D 792		Density (specific gravity)
D 1577	A	Linear density of textile fibers (denier)
D 2256	A-1	Breaking strength and elongation
		FABRIC
D 418		Pile fiber construction
D 418		Pile height (tuft height)
D 1335		Resistance to tuft pullout
D 1682	G-T	Grab tear strength
D 4158		Abrasion resistance (Uniform Abrasion Method)
D 2859		Flammability of pile floor covering (Methenamine Pill Test)
E 648		Flammability of synthetic turf (Flooring Radiant Panel Test)
F 1015		Relative abrasiveness of synthetic turf surfaces
D 5251		Resistance to matting (Tetrapod Method)
		SHOCK ABSORBING PAD COMPONENT
D 395	B	Compression set under constant load
D 624	Die C	Tear resistance
D 1667	D	Compression resistance (Modified Method)
D 1876		T-Peel strength of secondary pad
D 2126		Hydrolytic stability
D 3574	E	Tensile and elongation
D 3936		Delamination strength of secondary backing
F 355	A	Shock absorbency of playing surface systems and materials
D 3575	L	Water absorption (% Weight Gain)
		TURF SYSTEMS
F 1015		Relative abrasiveness of synthetic turf surfaces
D 1667	D	Compression resistance (Modified Method)
F 355	A	Shock absorbency of playing surface systems
MTP 030		Sports shoe traction and traction differential (coefficient of friction)
DIN 18 035		Water permeability of synthetic turf systems
F 1551		Ball bounce, ball rebound

References to AstroTurf®[2] show the unique properties of the original artificial turf and knowledge of the turf as a result of developing and manufacturing the system with Monsanto Company for 25 years.

Pile Fiber

The pile fiber in a synthetic turf playing surface provides the wear and weather-resisting portion of the system in addition to the grasslike appearance. Pile fibers have been stabilized for resistance to heat and ultraviolet radiation, designed to balance drainage and cleaning properties, and colored with durable pigments suspended in the fiber during its manufacture.

[2] AstroTurf is a registered trademark of AstroTurf Industries, Inc.

Current products incorporate these properties in the pile fiber, as measured by the following test methods:

Melting Point—ASTM Test Methods for Determination of Relative Viscosity, Melting Point, and Moisture Content of Polyamide (D 789)

Melting point of the pile fiber is related to its composition, chemistry, and flammability properties. The minimum standard for melting point in the majority of fields with synthetic turf pile fiber is at least 250°C. The normal melting point for nylon 6,6 is in the range of 256°C, nylon 6 is 218°C and polypropylene is 160°C.

Density (Specific Gravity)—ASTM Test Methods for Density and Specific Gravity (Relative Density) of Plastics by Displacement (D 792)

The density of the fiber is related to its chemistry as well as its physical properties—low density materials provide good "cover" but may offer less strength. Higher density materials tend to be stronger, but require more weight of material per unit of area for the same amount of "cover" or "apparent value." The best performance is obtained with high density fibers. Tests of nylon 6,6 used for synthetic surfaces show a density of 1.14 g/cm^3, nylon 6 at 1.14, and polypropylene at 0.91.

Both the melting point and density of nylon 6,6 ribbon are set by the physics and chemistry of the material. The high melting point means that the fiber will hold up well under heavy athletic traffic and will be less affected by the heat of a dropped match or cigarette. Strength, durability, ease of cleaning, and resistance to weather are benefits of nylon 6,6 pile fiber.

Filament Size—ASTM Test Method for Linear Density (Denier) of Textile Fibers (D 1577)

The denier is a big factor in its texture, strength, drainage rate, resistance to weathering, and ease of cleaning. Deniers were tested ranging from normal carpet fibers up to the 1100 denier level. It was found that deniers in the middle of the range give the best balance of these properties.

The denier of AstroTurf pile ribbon exceeds 500 denier per filament (dpf), and typically averages 550 denier. Larger deniers tend to be more abrasive or difficult to extrude, knit or tuft. (Denier is the weight in grams of a single yarn filament 9000 m long).

Breaking Strength and Elongation—ASTM Test Method for Tensile Properties of Yarns by the Single Strand Method (D 2256)

The tensile properties of fibers are a direct measure of their strength and how far fibers will stretch before breaking. The stronger the fiber and the more elastic, the better it will resist wear.

The breaking strength for pile fibers should exceed 3.0 g/denier. Typical production data should average 3.5 g/denier.

The breaking elongation is an indication of elasticity and resilience of the fiber should the elongation exceed 25% to meet ASTM Test Method D 2256. Typical production data for ribbon should average 30% elongation to break.

The combination of fiber polymer type, filament size, and tensile properties in nylon 6,6 fields gives the user the best balance of matting resistance, drainage, and wear and weather resistance. The aesthetic properties of a permanently pigmented, nonglare fiber stays attractive for years of heavy athletic usage. These properties are established by the physics in extrusion of fibers used in synthetic turf.

Pile Fabrics

Experience shows that the integrity of the fabric component of the playing surface system is a vital element in the performance of the total system. The properties listed below are the ones regarded as most important for surfaces used for heavy-duty athletic fields.

Construction—ASTM Test Methods of Testing Pile Yarn Floor Covering Construction (D 418)

Synthetic turfs are made by a number of manufacturing methods. Weaving is the traditional method, and was used for early AstroTurf surfaces. It is now seldom used because of its slow production rates and high costs. Tufting is the most common method of carpet manufacture today. Tufting can be less expensive and faster, but tufted turf is limited in strength, tuft bind, and resistance to rips and tears.

The knitting process produces fabrics as strong and durable as woven ones, but more resistant to wrinkles and puckers. Knitting requires specially modified equipment to handle the sizes and weights of fabric for synthetic turf playing fields.

In designing fabrics, a number of balances must be struck. If the surface pile is too sparse, wear and weather resistance are affected. Pile fiber that is packed too tightly will be abrasive and harsh, difficult to clean, and will drain slowly.

AstroTurf fabric is knitted, using all synthetic materials, with a pile fiber content exceeding 50 oz/yd^2 (1.7 kg/m^2). The backing fabric weighs 8.0 oz/yd^2 (0.27 kg/m^2), and the fabric contains 3.0 oz/yd^2 (0.10 kg/m^2) of precoat resin, for a total weight of 61 oz/yd^2 (2.0 kg/m^2). Lower weight fabrics can be produced, but usually cannot provide the performance requirements for weathering and wearing needed for outdoor fields.

Pile Height—ASTM Test Methods (D 418)

The pile height of a fabric should be great enough to provide good "cover," minimize "brushiness," give good wear resistance, but not so great that drainage is retarded excessively, cleaning made more difficult and traffic patterning more apparent. Pile heights between 0.50 and 0.75 in. (1.2 and 1.9 cm) appear to balance these properties well. The nominal pile height for stadium surface is (1.2 cm) $^1/_2$ in. or higher. Shorter pile fabrics tend to become more abrasive to players.

Resistance to Tuft Pullout—ASTM Test Method for Tuft Bind of Pile Floor Coverings (D 1335)

The tufts should be securely attached to the backing fabric, requiring at least 25 lb (11 kg) force to pull them out. Reports from independent test laboratories have shown tuft-bind values of above 25 to 30 lb (11 to 13 kg) for knitted nylon 6,6 surfaces. Actually, tuft failure in this test with knitted fabrics includes destruction of the backing yarns.

Tuft bind of tufted surfaces should exceed 8 lb (3.6 kg).

Grab Tear Strength—ASTM Test Method for Breaking Strength and Elongation of Textile Fabrics (D 5034)

The "grab tear strength" method measures the tear resistance of the total fabric structure rather than the strength of the fabric components taken independently. The grab tear strength of recreational surface fabrics should average at least 350 lb (158 kg) when tested both along and across the fabric.

Knitted nylon 6,6 fabrics are more resistant to damage from rips and tears than lower strength materials. Tests of surfaces in laboratories have frequently run above 385 lb (174 kg).

The combination of materials used, the construction, exceptional fabric strength and exceptional tuft-bind properties of knitted fabric means that knitted fields resist rips, tears, and mechanical damage better than any other synthetic turf. The knitting design used gives a fabric that is manageable and can be securely bonded to the underpad.

Abrasion Resistance—ASTM Test Method for Abrasion Resistance of Textile Fabrics (Uniform Abrasion Method) (D 4158)

The correlation between laboratory abrasion tests and field performance is affected by many factors not found in the laboratory, including soilage, air pollution, and types of traffic found in the field (e.g., baseball spikes versus multicleated soccer shoes).

Tests for abrasion resistance should ensure, however, the fabric system fall in the "highly resistant to abrasion" category. The "Uniform Abrasion Method" gives a good basis for making this judgment. Surfaces should lose less than 0.05 g from the abraded area of 50.8 mm^2 (2 in.^{2}) when subjected to 1000 cycles of the spring steel blade abradant under a 4.54-kg (10-lb) load. When nylon 6,6 surfaces are subjected to this test, the weight loss is usually less than 0.01 g.

Note: ASTM test methods for abrasion resistance all contain warnings against using them to compare textile materials having different types of fiber or different construction, unless the test in question has been validated by correlation with wear data from actual usage.

Synthetic turf surface fabric design has evolved through years of testing and development to give a proven record of exceptional strength, durability, and performance in heavy athletic field usage.

Flammability—ASTM Test Method for Flammability of Finished Textile Floor Covering Materials (D 2859)

This test determines the flammability of textile floor covering using the methenamine tablet method in a draft-protected environment by measuring the resulting char length.

This test method is used for measuring and describing the properties of materials in response to heat and flame under controlled laboratory conditions. It is considered as the "minimum" standard for indoor carpet and outdoor turf surfaces.

Fabric Flammability—ASTM Test Method for Critical Radiant Flux of Floor Covering Systems Using a Radiant Heat Energy Source (D 648)

Artificial turf surfaces are exposed to abuse both from carelessly dropped cigarettes and deliberate acts of vandalism. Knitted nylon 6,6 surfaces have an excellent record against both kinds of events. The flooring radiant panel method tests the heat flux required to maintain combustion in a floor covering, reporting it as "critical radiant flux" in watts per square centimeter.

Synthetic turf should have critical radiant flux values in excess of 0.35 W/cm^2. Independent laboratory results can range from 0.35 to 1.05+ W/cm^2. Knitted nylon 6,6 fabrics are less likely to be severely damaged by the heat or fire from dropped matches, cigarettes, or even the attacks of vandalism than synthetic turfs made of other materials or by other methods.

Resistance to Matting—ASTM Practice for the Operation of the Tetrapod Walker Drum Tester (D 5251)

This practice describes the equipment and operation of the Tetrapod Walker in matting and crushing of pile fabrics. Synthetic turfs should indicate their resistance to matting when tested comparatively in the tetrapod walker.

Nylon 6,6 pile fibers have a higher resistance to matting than polypropylene under this test and in actual outdoor use.

Shock-Absorbing Pad Component

The shock-absorbing pad component in the surface system is designed to provide both comfort and cushioning properties for athletes. It must do so throughout the range of weather conditions likely to be encountered in athletic usage.

To meet these demands, a closed-cell synthetic foam of high mechanical strength that resists the loss of properties as a result of wear, mechanical abuse, and weather is usually used. Some current pad systems are thoroughly tested in a wide range of climates and uses, and have performed well even under occasional traffic of lightweight pneumatic-tired motor vehicles normally found at athletic fields.

Compression Set Under Constant Load—ASTM Test Methods for Rubber Property—Compression Set (D 395)

For full usefulness of a playing field, it is sometimes necessary to erect temporary stands, drive vehicles on the field, or otherwise put loads on the surface for hours, days, or even longer. This compressive set test measures the loss of pad thickness following exposure to a constant load of 45.36 kg/m^2 (100 lb/in.^{2}) for a period of 22 h, and a 24 h recovery period, both at standard laboratory temperature and humidity of 21 to 24°C (70 to 75°F) and 60 to 65% relative humidity (RH).

High permanent set values for closed cell pads suggest poor durability or performance. Pads used for football surfaces normally have 20 to 30% set under this severe test.

Tear Resistance—ASTM Test Method for Tear Strength of Conventional Vulcanized Rubber and Thermoplastic Elastomers (D 624)

This test is a characterization of rubber or foam samples by tear resistance. The sample is a 90° angle specimen cut with ASTM Die C. The minimum tear strength of the shock-absorbing pad component is 9.1 kg (20 lb) by this test method.

Compression Resistance—ASTM Specification for Flexible Cellular Materials—Vinyl Chloride Polymers and Copolymers (Closed-Cell Form) (D 1667)

This test measures the force required to compress the pad to 75% of its original thickness (25% compression). Experience has shown that values between 3.18 and 4.5 kg/in.^{2} (7 and 10 lb/in.^{2}) provide for good player comfort values in most applications. Values for pad in most fields run at approximately 3.85 kg/in.^{2} (8.5 lb/in.^{2}) when tested at standard laboratory temperature and humidity.

The shock-absorbing pad component should be designed to give the best balance of "comfort" and "cushion" properties under the conditions encountered in heavy outdoor athletic usage.

T-Peel Strength of Secondary Pad—ASTM Test Method for Peel Resistance of Adhesives (D 1876)

Peel strength should exceed 3.63 kg/in. (8 lb/in.) and typically is stronger than the shock-absorbing pad component. It is extremely important that the peel strength does not deteriorate significantly in submerged water tests, in environmental aging, or in field use.

Stability to Heat and Moisture—ASTM Test Method for Response of Rigid Cellular Plastics to Thermal and Humid Aging (D 2126)

Most closed-cell foam systems tend to lose their properties through gas diffusion from the cells under hot, wet conditions. Exposure of the pad to 65.6°C (150°F) and 98% RH for 28 days will indicate the tendency for gas loss in service. Do not consider pad systems that lose more than 25% of their volume following such exposures as acceptable. Typical values from independent laboratory tests for closed-cell pads show volume losses of only 4 to 5% following 28-day environmental aging.

The pad system used under surfaces can take the loads required for many different activities, both static and moving. Synthetic turf systems are truly multiple-use facilities. Their ability to withstand outdoor exposure has been proven both in the laboratory and in actual field service.

Tensile and Elongation Properties—ASTM Test Methods for Vulcanized Rubber and Thermoplastic Rubbers and Thermoplastic Elastomers–Tension (D 412)

Low mechanical strength makes the pad subject to delamination and tearing in service. Tests show that, for good performance, the pads used under heavy-duty athletic fields should have tensile strengths exceeding 40.8 kg/in.^{2} (90 lb/in.^{2}) and breaking elongations above 125%. Typical values for the pad used under fields run 52 kg/in.^{2} (115 lb/in.^{2}) breaking strength and 130% elongation to break.

Delamination Strength of Secondary Backing—ASTM Test Method for Delamination Strength of Secondary Backing of Pile Floor Coverings (D 3936)

Secondary backings are added to carpeting and synthetic turf fabrics to improve the durability, dimensional stability, and other properties desired for installing the products. Therefore, the adherence strength of the secondary to the turf must be strong enough to withstand the severe traffic and environmental conditions. Strength of the laminant should be as follows:

Target—6.8 kg/in. (15 lb/in.)

Minimum—4.5 kg/in. (10 lb/in.)

Range—4.5 to 9 kg/in. (10 to 20 lb/in.)

Shock Attenuation of Shock Absorbing-Pad Component—ASTM Test Method for Shock-Absorbing Properties of Playing Surface Systems and Materials (F 355)

Shock attenuation of a playing surface is highly dependent on the shock-absorbing properties of the pad component and/or base in installations containing an "elastic layer."

Either one of the components can be checked for its shock-absorbing properties in the laboratory or field using Procedure A of ASTM Test Method F 355. An impact velocity of 3.43 ± 0.17 m/s is required. The velocity corresponds to a theoretical drop height of 0.61 m (24 in.) at sea level. A uniaxial accelerometer in or on the missile is used to monitor the acceleration-time history of the impact. G is the ratio of the magnitude of missile acceleration during impact to the acceleration of gravity, and G_{max} is the Maximum Value of G encountered during impact.

Shock-absorbing "undercushions" used in current football fields can range from 75 to 130 G_{max}. Pad systems over 100 G_{max} should be avoided.

Water Absorption—ASTM Test Methods for Flexible Cellular Materials Made from Olefin Polymers (D 3575)

The open cell content of shock-absorbing pad components affects the firmness and shock-absorbing properties of the system when wet or frozen.

The shock-absorbing pad component should absorb less than 3% water on a weight basis, although ASTM Test Method D 3575 calls for reporting the water absorption expressed in kilograms/metre of cut surface area.

Turf Systems

Relative Abrasiveness—ASTM Test Method for Relative Abrasiveness of Synthetic Turf Playing Surfaces (F 1015)

Resistance to abrasive wear and minimal abrasiveness to players' apparel, and equipment tend to oppose each other. ASTM Test Method F 1015 measures the ability of a synthetic turf surface to wear away a standard synthetic polymer foam during sliding weighted contact and correlates well with both subjective and other objective measures of abrasiveness.

Surfaces typically should show Abrasiveness Index values of less than 40 under standard laboratory conditions. Typical range for synthetic turfs is 30 to 60.

Compressive Resistance (Modified Method)—ASTM Specification for Flexible Cellular Materials—Vinyl Chloride Polymers and Copolymers (Closed Cell Form) (D 1667)

An indention force deflection (IDF) test can be made on system samples using a 2.87-cm (1.129-in. diameter) compressive foot or ram to compress the sample in measuring the compressive resistance or "softness" of the system.

Compression of the sample can be deflected to 25 or 37.5% of its original thickness, immediately recording the force required at 25% deflection in thickness. The compressive resistance of a system will be higher than the shock pad alone because of the load spreading of the fabric surface and the test method used.

Shock Absorbency of Playing Surface Systems—ASTM Test Method for Shock-Absorbing Properties of Playing Surface Systems and Materials (F 355)

"Softness," "hardness," and "comfort" are difficult to measure by any single test. "Shock absorbency" is the ability of a playing surface to spread out the time and lessen the force of a blow or fall onto a playing surface. The referenced test requires dropping a heavy weight missile onto the playing surface and using electronic equipment to record how the surface absorbs the impact.

Procedure A of the above test method is used to test synthetic turf football and baseball systems. Newly manufactured samples of stadium surface systems test below 100 G_{max}, typically 75 G_{max} when tested at 21 to 24°C (70 to 75°F) and 60 to 65% relative humidity. Soccer fields are tested by the same method, but the shock attenuation typically exceeds 200 G_{max}.

TABLE 2—*Shock attenuation of football fields.*

	Desired G_{max}	Typical Range
New fields	$< 100\ G_{max}$	75 to 125 G_{max}
Old fields	$< 150\ G_{max}$	75 to 350 G_{max}
Suggested maximum: 225 G_{max}		

An impact velocity of 3.43 ± 0.17 m/s is required for this test method. This velocity corresponds to a theoretical drop height of 0.61 m (24 in.) at sea level. A uniaxial accelerometer in or on the missile is used to monitor the acceleration-time history of the impact.

Turf systems show change in impact values when tested at pad temperatures as low as 0°C (32°F) or as high as 49°C (120°F).

The technology and materials are available so that synthetic or natural turf football and baseball systems should not exceed 225 G_{max} when properly engineered and maintained. Shock attenuation of football fields is shown in Table 2.

Sports Shoe Traction and Traction Differential—Synthetic Turf Traction (Coefficient of Friction) AT-030

The shoe characteristics and surface properties significantly affect the traction. This method is used to measure the traction (coefficient of friction) between shoes and playing surfaces. Traction is the force required to initiate or maintain movement in a weighted sports shoe on a playing surface divided by the vertical loading force of the shoe plus the added weights.

Morehouse [1] reported the basic mechanism that results in many lower extremity joint injuries, according to most medical experts, is that the foot becomes fixed as a result of excessive traction and the shoe becomes "locked" into the turf when changing directions or result from contact with other players.

Hamner and Orofino [2] reported measuring the coefficient of static friction between the playing surface and the shoe determines the traction and the shoe characteristics significantly affect the traction. Therefore, this test method can be used to measure the traction of different turfs with a "standard" shoe or different shoes on the same turf.

Valiant [3] reported the minimum traction needs of a soccer shoe on artificial turf should have a coefficient of friction of 0.8 or greater when forces are exerted in an anterior direction, and 0.6 when forces are exerted in a lateral direction.

Until more refined tests are adopted, this method can be used to more closely match the shoe to the football surface in laboratory and actual field testing. Outdoor surfaces should be checked when wet and when dry. It appears from the limited data available, that the shoe traction (ST) is as approximated below.

Desired ST—0.8 to 1.2

Actual range—0.4 to 2.5*

*Actual field data would be required to confirm actual field shoe traction range.

Water Permeability of Synthetic Turf Systems—Water Permeability of Synthetic Turf and Permeable Bases (DIN 18-035)

Some exciting developments have been accomplished in turf drainage and permeability in recent years. These range from systems to remove the maximum amount of water during a downpour of rain, to removing excess water but leaving the turf wet, all just to improve the game of play or extend it to completion with minimum delays.

The referenced method was originally designed to audit the porosity of asphalt, concrete, and rubber bases before turf was installed. It was later refined to check the drainage rate of most turf covered football, baseball, hockey, and soccer fields or systems.

Typical water permeability of synthetic turf systems and permeable bases are:

Football/Baseball—25 to 100 cm/h (10 to 40 in./h)   (rain-fall capacity)

Hockey/Soccer—15 cm/h (6 in./h)   (FIH minimum rate)

Turf System Ball Bounce, Ball Rebound

This test method addresses only the basic, and useful, sports ball and playing surface interaction of the coefficient of restitution on vertical impingement. Typical values for each sport are in Table 3.

Installation

Seams and joints in synthetic turf systems represent potential weak spots for wear and vandalism and should be minimized. All surfaces should be installed by experienced crews using materials suitable for the climate of the installation site and for the designed uses of the installation.

Seam Frequency

• Side seams in the fabric are at 15-ft intervals, matching the 5-yd lines on a typical football field. Fewer seams means less chance for problems.
• All seams are sewn with a double-locked stitch to give strength and durability.
• There are no "head" or "butt" seams on the playing surface for normal football/soccer fields.

System Bonding

• The underpad is installed over the asphalt substrate in a uniform manner with no visible bubbles or areas that show up as "soft spots" or water traps.
• The fabric is bonded to the underpad with no visible wrinkles, ripples, or bubbles. If any such bubbles occur, they are repaired by the installers in such a way that the strength of the fabric system is not impaired. Avoid slitting the surface fabric to relieve wrinkles. Reinforce and repair any slits.

TABLE 3—*Typical values for baseball, hockey, and soccer.*

Sport	Height, m	Desired Rebound, %	Range, %
Baseball	2	20	15 to 25
	5		
Hockey	1.5	15	8 to 20
Soccer	3	24	20 to 28

Painting

Fields are painted with the markings required for the principal game to be played. Use paint materials that are compatible with the turf, give good resistance to the wear of game traffic, and good visibility for players, officials, and spectators.

Significance

No synthetic turf is better than the job done in its installation. Fields should be well made, carefully installed, and supported by a full-time, year-round professional service organization, with the experience of installing playing fields worldwide.

Conclusion

The test methods and performance criteria described in this paper for synthetic turf surfaces serve as benchmarks for characterizing and communicating properties of artificial turf. The American Society for Testing and Materials (ASTM) procedures and test methods described herein should be used to establish the minimum standards and properties of synthetic turf components and systems.

References

[1] Morehouse, C. A., "Artificial Turf," *Turfgrass—Agronomy Monograph 32* ASA-CSSA-SSSA, 677S Segoe Rd., Madison, WI 53711, 1992.

[2] Hamner, W. F. and Orofino, T. A., "Recreational Surfaces," *Encyclopedia of Chemistry and Technology*, Vol. 19, 3rd ed., In Kirk-Othmer, Ed., John Wiley and Sons, New York, 1982, pp. 922–936.

[3] Valiant, G. A., "Traction Needs and Friction Characteristics of Athletic Footwear," NIKE, Inc., 900 S. W. Nimbus, Beaverton, OR 97005 (date unpublished).

David Dury[1] and John S. Craggs[2]

The Envelope System—Performance and Experience in the United Kingdom

REFERENCE: Dury, D. and Craggs, J. S. "**The Envelope System—Performance and Experience in the United Kingdom,**" *Safety in American Football, ASTM STP 1305,* Earl F. Hoerner, Ed., American Society for Testing and Materials, 1996, pp. 114–122.

ABSTRACT: The patented *envelope system* consists of a layer of specially selected sand or stone wrapped in a strong but highly porous membrane. This prevents erosion but allows moisture to pass through at a very high rate.

A high drainage rate has two major benefits. First, standing water is not a problem provided the surfacing material is porous to allow water into the base. Second, as little water remains within the base, the effects of frost heave are minimized.

The material in the envelope is selected so that particle size, shape, and distribution do not allow over compaction or settling out. As a result, the playing characteristics and drainage capabilities are maintained over a long period. Since 1981, experience in the United Kingdom has shown that the system matures the longer it has been down.

The special geotextile "Nottsfilm" that encases the sand or stone, has been especially developed to allow for high porosity and enable particulate material to be retained. It is a resin-bonded, needle-punched, polyester fabric only 1 to 2 mm thick yet its load-bearing capabilities are so good that only one layer is normally required. The pore spaces in the material are evenly distributed, thus, giving consistent drainage throughout the material.

By using natural particulate materials as the base, construction is similar to a natural turf pitch with a synthetic turf surface. This combination results in playing characteristics close to those of natural turf being achieved on an installation with the usage capabilities of synthetic turf. Tests carried out in United Kingdom meet the requirements of the Winterbottom report for soccer pitches.

Injuries associated with synthetic turf areas consist primarily of either stress-related injuries to the limbs or friction burns. On conventionally constructed engineered bases, it is very difficult to eliminate these factors, as solid base construction contributes to both injuries. The *envelope system* is better on both counts. First, the natural impact absorption properties mean that the stresses caused by interactions with the surface are similar to those exhibited by natural turf pitches. Second, the possibility and degree of friction burns are reduced because much of the energy is dissipated into the air spaces between the materials in the base leaving less energy available to be turned into heat.

KEYWORDS: sports field base construction, synthetic turf, injury prevention, envelope system, dynamic bases, unbound structures

This paper and presentation to the symposium on Safety in American Football is a summary of over 20 years research and experience in the development of synthetic turf systems and surfaces for sport and recreation. The findings have been greatly influenced by the work of Peter L. K. Dury, father of the coauthor. He was the original "inventor" of the "envelope" system.

[1] Export manager, Notts Sport, Launde House, Harborough Rd, Oadby, Leicester, LE2 4LE, England.
[2] Managing director, Safety Play Systems Inc., P.O. Box 4124, Victoria, B.C. V8X 3X4, Canada.

In the early years of development of synthetics in many countries, the emphasis was on the carpet surface. Very few people paid much attention to the base that the carpet was laid upon, and the criterion was that it was "all weather" and a true, flat surface.

Carpet technology has progressed enormously in the past 20 years, with the introduction of hard-wearing carpets, pile configurations that give greater grip and traction to the athlete, whatever sport is being played, and the introduction of better jointing methods.

The use of sand-filled carpets to reduce costs, but maintain wearability, can in fact have other attributes such as less heat friction, but conversely give more abrasion from the sand.

The introduction of special fibers for the pile of the surface, the change from nylon to polypropylene yarns, and the use of specially coated fibers to reduce friction in certain circumstances, known as low slip resistant (LSR) fibers, have all proven to be important factors in the development of the synthetic turf surfaces.

Effect of the Base Under the Carpet

It was recognized from an early stage that a shockpad or shock layer for most sports was required and these sometimes were introduced as part of the carpet backing. The rest were introduced as rubber or foam underlays laid as a separate sheet or in a poured-in-place format. The majority of which are still, even with today's developments, laid on a bitumen-bound base structure or interlocking stone to dust with a wide particle range to give what is believed to be a stable base structure.

In 1969, Peter Dury (and in subsequent years Notts Sport) approached the provision of a sports facility in a completely reverse order compared to the majority of people in the industry. He considered the base structure first.

As a professionally trained groundsman, he looked at the aggregates used within the subbase, and, using his knowledge of soil technology, realized that stability is dependent upon the size, shape, and distribution of the particles and their interlocking properties. The common factors that influence all sports surfaces, synthetic and natural, are water, air, the size and shape of the particles used in the structure, and the ability of the structure to remain stable, but not rigid. To create quality and good value for sports facilities, research for schools over the next ten years in Nottinghamshire County resulted in a range of patented products and designs with potential applications worldwide.

The use of loose or nonbonded-base structures had been recognized by a number of people. In particular, in the United Kingdom, the experience of a European neighbor, Holland, had an influence on the use of what are commonly known today as *dynamic* bases. This created a dilemma for many facility providers. Do we go "bound" base, which is commonly termed *engineered,* or do we go "unbound," *dynamic?*

However, some of the early dynamic pitches installed by certain companies did not do justice to this particular method of construction. As a result of the wide range of particles in the structure, some constructions eventually became just as hard as a bound base, and on occasions, had no supplementary shock layer. Others, because of inadequate porosity, moved when frost caused uneven expansion of the structure. This hindered the acceptance of dynamic bases for a number of years. In an effort to create a stable base structure, the main criteria that appeared to have been overlooked were particle shape, size, and its effect on play.

During the early 1980s at Nottinghamshire County Council, extensive research and experience with synthetic turf cricket pitches took place. These pitches required the ball to bounce on impact with the surface in a very uniform manner and also to have changes in the way the pitch played, depending on moisture and compaction to simulate natural turf. Some of the first multipurpose games and children's playgrounds were installed in schools. These areas

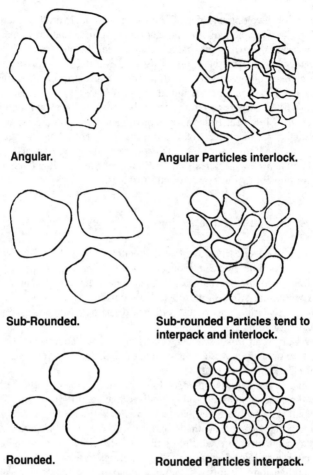

Angular.   Angular Particles interlock.

Sub-Rounded.   Sub-rounded Particles tend to
                           interpack and interlock.

Rounded.   Rounded Particles interpack.

FIG. 1—*Particle shape.*

used different sized particles within the base structure to give different levels of ball bounce or shock absorbency depending on the particular application.

The results that followed indicated that the particle size and shape were as important as the distribution of the particles (Fig. 1). Not only would high ball bounce and consequent high energy return be experienced with a wide range of particles, interlocking to form a rigid base, but also if angular particles were used this would also give a higher ball bounce. Tests were carried out on areas using the same size particles, with one area using rounded particles and the other angular but both having the same distribution of particle sizes.[3]

On the rounded particles, low bounce was experienced and on the angular particles high ball bounce (Fig. 2). This is due to the movement of the particles within the structure (Fig. 3). Very fluid particles, of course, tended to create disturbance from the surface and so totally

[3] "To Play Like Natural Turf." This report was based on an investigation into the use of particulate and synthetic materials in the provision of sports facility base formations, using grant aid from the Football Trust and the Sports Council in the United Kingdom for the installation of protype pitches.

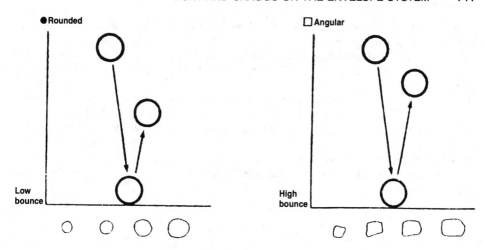

Distribution and size identical.

FIG. 2—*A narrow range of particles.*

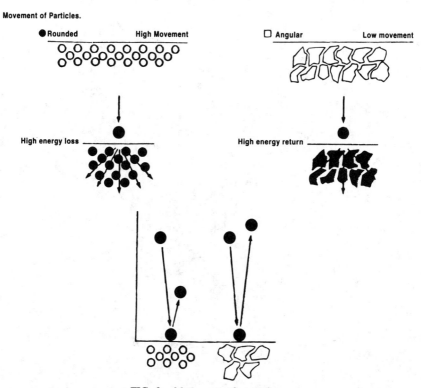

FIG. 3—*Movement of particles.*

rounded particles were only practical in a fully mobile surface, i.e., in children's playgrounds as a means of absorbing energy.

For sports areas, a balance was required and so particles were used that were of a subrounded nature to allow pivotability and not full fluid movement. The particles were allowed to interpack (Figs. 4 and 5).

The other factor to take into consideration was dependent on what size ball was to impact on the surface and to determine how much influence the size of the particle had on the bounce of the ball. Choosing smaller particles could create lower bounce and yet still feel firm provided not too wide a range was used (Fig. 6). So by choosing a balance of particles both in size, shape, and distribution, a stable base structure can be created, giving the feeling of a firm structure as provided by large interlocking particles or a wide range of particles, yet with less ball bounce and consequently less reflection of energy.

● **Pivotability.**
Moves about in contact with surrounding particles.

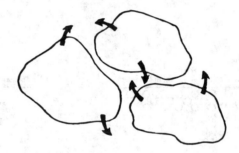

● **Fluidity**
Moves Freely

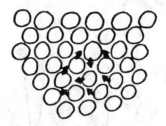

Key.... Direction of Movement.

FIG. 4—*Pivotability and fluidity of particles.*

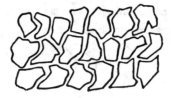

● **Interlocking.**

Holds together firmly, within each other due to the shape of the particles.

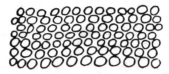

● **Interpacking.**

Holds together without interlocking due to the volume of materials within the space. Interpacking particles tend to be fluid and have pivotability.

FIG. 5—*Interlocking and interpacking of particles.*

Use of Geotextiles

Additional research in Nottinghamshire involved the use of geotextiles within the construction that had been introduced to separate different layers of aggregates. Coupled with the knowledge of how different particle sizes and shapes influence the performance of a ball or athlete on impact, the "envelope system" was created.

The patented "envelope" shockpad system consists of an unbound particulate layer, either carefully selected sand or clean stone, enclosed by a highly porous fiber-bonded textile, called "Nottsfilm." This structure can be laid onto existing foundations or a suitably designed and constructed foundation and drainage system applicable to the particular site conditions.

The "envelope" method of isolating the particulate layers means that much finer and more refined particles can be selected without fear of erosion or contamination by the lower layers of foundation stone. With other methods of construction, using unbounded materials, the materials selected for each layer of buildup need to hold together to prevent migration of particles from one layer to another. This can result in a form of structure that even with the addition of shockpads can feel hard to the user on high impact.

"Nottsfilm" is used as the isolating layer in preference to other less expensive geotextiles. Its method of manufacture using the needle-punched process provides a more even permeability than with spun woven fabrics that can have areas that are denser than others. The uniform porosity is very important to avoid hazards that have been minimized by careful particle selection. Additionally, unlike other needle-punched fabrics, "Nottsfilm" has a resin impregnation to bind the fibers and give greater strength and load-bearing qualities.

(A) Bounce of a small sphere on large particles.
Large particles interlocking loosely.

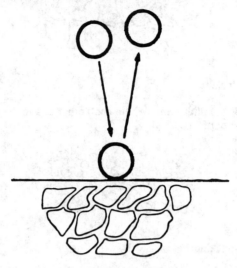

(B) Bounce of a small sphere on small particles.
Small particles interlocking to the same extent as in (A).

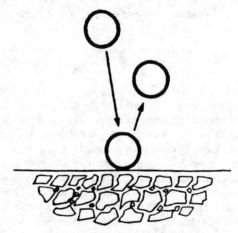

FIG. 6—*Bounce of small sphere.*

The Envelope System and Increased Safety

First we must consider the relationship between sports and common factors in playing performance.

Field hockey—The main sport around which synthetic pitches in Europe have been developed. Ball rebound, ball roll, ball deviation, permeability, surface friction, ball/surface friction, force reduction, and, at a later date, peak G have been the main criteria.

Soccer—Ball rebound, velocity change, traction, sliding distance, and peak G are the major criteria.

American football—Peak G, surface friction, and traction are the major criteria.

The most common factor for all sports is energy absorption. Although, in many cases, we still find many people wishing to install nonturf sports facilities who treat this aspect as a minor concern and not a major factor. Their main priority in these cases is the test methods relating to ball performance. We believe energy absorption is one of the most important considerations.

As with test methods for a number of sports, the concerns of the players after some years of experience with synthetics can also show common factors.

Concerns Regarding Synthetic Surfaces

American football—Injuries to players.

Soccer—Injuries to players and high ball bounce, hence the decision of the professional Soccer Association in the United Kingdom to ban the use of all synthetic pitches for league play.

Field hockey—Injuries to players, in particular stress-related injuries. In many cases, these are not attributable to one particular impact, but what should also be considered is the increased overplay and training that synthetic pitches have allowed. Recently, the All England Women's Hockey Association (AEWHA) has started to investigate in more detail the etiology of injury.

In a recent paper, Carl Ward, Director of Coaching, AEWHA, stated:

> one aspect that is currently attracting increasing attention is the degree of player comfort and safety offered by these revolutionary surfaces. There is now growing concern in a number of sports that intensive play on inappropriate surfaces may be contributing to the number and variety of stress related injuries currently being experienced by sports people and athletes.
> With this in mind, many Governing Bodies of Sport have issued performance standards which give some idea of what is "acceptable" as a sports pitch. Hockey is no exception and I would urge all specifiers to scrutinize these guidelines, select those which will provide you with a desired level of performance and comfort and then decide on the design which will provide and deliver this.

All these concerns have become a major issue even with the availability of many shockpad layers on the market today.

Designers have attempted to reduce the harmful effects of a person or a ball coming into contact with the pitch by introducing a rubber crumb or similar shockpad between the solid base formation and the synthetic surface. On conventionally constructed engineered bases, it is very difficult to eliminate these problems because the solid base construction contributes to both these factors. The pitch does not yield to the pressures exerted when a player runs and turns, so all the stresses are focused on the player's limbs. On a natural turf pitch, the surface gives and some energy is lost into the structure, thus, lowering the stress on the player.

On particulate- or dynamic-based installations the actual particulate materials with careful selection have the ability to absorb a great deal of the impact throughout their entire structure.

The methods of test for Peak G in relation to soccer and field hockey in the United Kingdom are measured from a drop height of only 1 or 1.5 m. Many of the elastic layers on bound bases pass these tests without too much difficulty.

The question we would like to raise is—should the whole structure be shock absorbent?

The experience in the United Kingdom in using particulate-base formations on children's playgrounds indicated that energy from greater heights penetrates the structure deeper and so the subbase on which the energy absorption layer is laid starts to have a greater influence. With the same shockpad laid on a base formation, including asphalt or concrete, the shockpad may "bottom out" when a given weight falls from a specific height.[4]

---

[4] Technical Report CTR 11833, dated 26 March 1986, produced by RAPRA Technology Ltd. for Nottinghamshire County Council.

In other words, the shock absorbent material is compressed to such an extent that the energy penetrates to the solid base formation rather than being absorbed within the shockpad. Under such circumstances, although the structure may feel soft on impact, there may well be secondary effects. This would apply particularly to the bonded rubber materials, as the elasticity of the pad in returning to its original form may set up secondary shock waves back into the anatomy of the athlete. This would suggest that a safer option would be to have a structure that absorbs energy throughout the entire structure with minimal reflection.

We believe quality-dynamic bases offer this possibility. The "envelope system" offers a quality-dynamic base, with the structural stability to avoid the problems associated with many other unbound structures.

The "envelope," combined with other underlays such as fiber stabilized shockpads, when applicable, offers a range of facilities from children's playgrounds (very shock absorbent) to cricket pitches (fairly hard to reflect energy), with many other sports coming somewhere between.

Conclusion

We feel that American football, along with other field sports, in the United States, should carefully consider the "envelope system" technology within their designs both for player comfort and increased safety.

Reference

[1]   Dury, P. K. and Dury, P., Jr., "To Play Like Natural Turf," Nottinghamshire County Council, 1985.

Patrick M. Gorham[1] and T. A. Orofino[1]

Actual Field Performance of Synthetic Turf as Measured over a Thirty Year Period

REFERENCE: Gorham, P. M. and Orofino, T. A., "**Actual Field Performance of Synthetic Turf as Measured over a Thirty Year Period,**" *Safety in American Football, ASTM STP 1305,* Earl F. Hoerner, Ed., American Society for Testing and Materials, 1996, pp. 123–131.

ABSTRACT: Over the past 30 years, AstroTurf® Manufacturing, Inc. has performed field inspections of various synthetic turf fields throughout the U.S. Testing included turf color retention, fiber wear, turf performance, padding system performance, pavement performance, as well as the subbases. To date, over 250 fields have been tested. Testing has been performed at various times of the year with recorded weather conditions, i.e., temperature, humidity, and rainfall.

Along with the visual inspections, various physical properties of the turf system have been tested by trained technicians. Pile height retention, shoe traction, turf friction, and G_{max} were made. This paper will focus on the G_{max} testing (ASTM Test Method for Shock-Absorbing Properties of Play Surface and Materials F 355, Procedure A) over this 30 year period. This field test data will be compared with "laboratory accelerated wear" testing performed on turf and pad. This will also illustrate the correlation between accelerated lab testing of turf products to "real live" testing.

The G_{max} values will be broken down further into various subcategories:

(A) G_{max} values versus the life of fields. This will show the progression or loss of shock absorbency of the total field as the years of wear and use occur.

(B) G_{max} values versus padding systems. This will show the evolution of pad systems. Improved performance and longevity, as well as player comfort of pad systems after years of development and testing indication.

(C) G_{max} progression (increase) of specific fields. This will chart how individual field G_{max} values progress over time. Several fields will be examined, and a relationship drawn between life of the field and amount of usage versus G_{max} values.

KEYWORDS: G_{max}, athletic surfaces, AstroTurf synthetic playing surfaces, artificial turf, shock absorbency

Over the past 30 years, AstroTurf® Manufacturing Inc. has performed field inspections and testing of various synthetic turf fields throughout the U.S. Testing included turf color retention, fiber wear, turf performance, pad system, and subbase performance. Over 250 fields have been impact tested to date, at various times of the year, with recording of weather conditions, such as air temperature, humidity, and recent rainfall history. Along with the visual inspections, various physical properties of the turf system have been measured by trained technicians, either on the field or subsequently in the laboratory. Typical tests included pile height retention, shoe traction, turf friction, and G_{max}. Quantitative test data in this paper will focus primarily on the shock attenuation (G_{max}) testing (ASTM Test Method for Shock-Absorbing Properties

[1]Technical manager and consultant, respectively, AstroTurf® Manufacturing, Inc., 809 Kenner St., Dalton, GA 30721.

of Play Surface and Materials (F 355) Procedure A) over this period. The G_{max} values will be broken down further into various subcategories, including: G_{max} versus pad type, location on the field, ambient temperature, and field age. Astro Turf fields used for American football are the principal considerations.

General Consideration of System Performance Requirements

Turf Performance

Shoe Traction

The test method [1] used by AstroTurf to measure static and sliding shoe traction is the dragging of a weighted sports shoe across the turf surface. Measurements of the forces needed both to initiate and maintain motion are made. The resulting value for static or sliding friction is obtained by dividing the pulling force by the combined weight of the shoe and shoe load.

Shoe traction data from field inspections are relatively limited at this time. Typical values for recent Astro Turf, texturized nylon turf fields are indicated in Table 1. We should note that there are many aspects of shoe traction beyond the scope of this paper. A significant amount of research has been done by shoe manufacturers and the academic community. Work continues in this area as we try to work with these groups to produce the most meaningful research results.

Turf Pile Height

Pile height is defined as the height of pile measured from the surface of the backing to the tips of the pile fibers. ASTM Methods of Testing Woven and Tufted Pile Floor Covering (D 418). The pile height of AstroTurf products is a nominal 0.5 in. (13 mm). This optimum was derived from consideration of many factors, including shoe traction, player comfort, ball-turf interaction, and G_{max} reduction.

In indoor installations, the pile height remains relatively the same throughout the life cycle of the product, allowing for no noticeable differences in playing parameters. On outdoor installations, especially in high ultraviolet and humidity regions of the world, there is a very gradual change in pile height, more apparent in the high traffic areas of the field. There are many factors that influence the rate of pile reduction, and there is no constant value that can be derived. The influences of weather, amount of use, maintenance, and pollution levels are large factors in pile retention. As with any playing surface, synthetic turf fields should be regularly inspected and tested to determine the performance and safety of the surface and the system.

Turf Durability and Playability

A natural grass field will withstand 50 to 100 h per year of hard usage in most climates, and, even then, requires constant maintenance to retain its quality. Some synthetic turf fields

TABLE 1—*Typical shoe friction values for Astroturf surfaces.*

Nylon 66 Turf (Texturized)	Coefficient of Static Friction	Coefficient of Sliding Friction
New turf	1.2 to 1.5	1.0 to 1.3
Exposed turf	0.9 to 1.2	0.8 to 1.1

Curve (a)
ORIGINAL PAD SYSTEM
ASTM F-355A Gmax CURVE

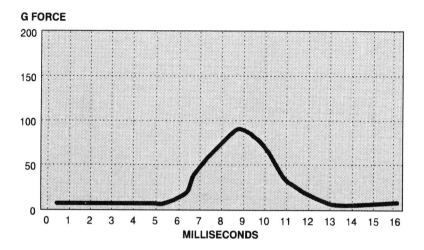

Curve (b)
OLD PAD SYSTEM
ASTM F-355A Gmax CURVE

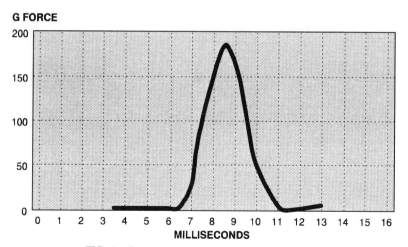

FIG. 1—*Representative curves from* G_{max} *testing.*

are used for up to 3500 h per year, and most are used for more than 2000 h per year in all climate extremes of hot, cold, humid, and arid areas [3].

The four major factors that affect the wear longevity of a synthetic turf surface are:

(1) exposure to ultraviolet radiation, present in sunlight;
(2) soilage from dust and dirt;
(3) wear from user traffic; and
(4) exposure to severe air pollution, including "acid rain."

Depending upon impact of the above listed factors, turf installations may wear at different rates. The turf performance should be monitored annually. As with most heavily used outdoor products, proper maintenance is essential to keep the surface in optimum playing condition. It is advised that the field maintenance persons follow the recommended maintenance procedures outlined in the owner's manual. Field aesthetics and performance can be greatly affected by the quality of the grounds crew.

Design of the turf itself continues to evolve and be fine tuned over the years. Significant changes such as textured turf have greatly improved uniformity of shoe traction and other performance indices. Several significant changes and the resulting improvements over a 30 year period are listed in Table 2.

Turf/Pad System Performance

Requirements

The three major factors that affect longevity of a shock-absorbing turf/pad system are:

(1) exposure to extreme heat and moisture,
(2) extreme wear from user traffic, and
(3) thickness retention of pad.

A good impact-absorbing system must exhibit hysteresis, converting some of the energy into nonrecoverable heat, not simply returning all of it as elastic rebound [1]. The recognized testing standard for measuring the shock absorbing playing surfaces is ASTM Test Method for Shock Absorbing Properties of Playing Surfaces Systems and Materials (F 355, Procedure A) and ASTM Standard Method for Comprehensive Characterization of Synthetic Turf Playing

TABLE 2—*Major design changes in Astroturf surfaces, 1964 to 1994.*

Turf Code	Design Feature	Principal Improvement
S 10	Woven construction	Original (Astrodome) Astroturf fabric
S 40	Tufted construction	Cost effective production methods
S 22	Knitted construction	Integrated, three-dimensional structure
S 34	Increase in pile weight (knitted)	Increased pile height and pile density for heavy-duty service
S 54	Textured pile ribbon* (knitted)	Textured pile-minimal directionality, reduced matting, decreased G_{max}, and sewn seams
S 65	Enhanced fiber denier (knitted)	Additional advance in pile face weight for longer life
SD 55	Enhanced fiber cross section	Longer playing life

*Orofino, T. A., *Polymer News,* Vol. 10, 1985, pp. 294–300.

Surfaces and Materials (F 1551). The test procedure uses the dropping of a 20 lb (9.1 kg), 20 in.^{2} (129 cm^2) cross-sectional area, flat missile equipped with a piezoelectric accelerometer that measures the G-forces generated throughout the impact event with the playing surface. Theoretically, the 20 lb missile approximates the weight of the human head and neck, and the 20 in.^{2}, the facial plane area of the human head. The missile is dropped from a 24 in. (61 cm) theoretical drop height, using an impact velocity of 136 in./s (345 cm/s). The acceleration or deceleration values were recorded against time via a digital oscilloscope. The peak of the curve is recorded as the G_{max}, and this value is generally reported as the index of performance for the turf/pad system. Additional G_{max} curve analyses that can be used are the "Severity Index" and the "Head Injury Criteria (HIC)" [3].

Shown below are examples of G_{max} curves representing two extremes of turf/pad performance. Curve (a) represents the performance of an original pad system in the 80 to 85 G_{max} range. Curve (b) represents a pad with a much higher G_{max} value, indicating that the pad system is near the end of its useful life.

AstroTurf engineered and developed its turf/pad system to impact between 80 and 90 G_{max} at installation. The pad has been designed to withstand the rigors placed upon it by most stadium uses.

Turf/Pad Versus Natural Grass

AstroTurf research impact tested many well-known and well-maintained grass fields. It was found that values ranged from G_{max} of 65 on muddy grass fields to as high as 275 in freezing conditions. There is obviously a high degree of variance in natural playing surfaces. Under the same conditions, AstroTurf tested between 75 and 150 G_{max} [2].

Temperature response of natural turf is minimal in short-term variation, but artificial surfaces do vary with pad temperature. The following chart (Fig. 2) shows the temperature response curve of the current turf and pad system.

Shock-Absorbing Pad Component Developments

During the past 30 years, continuous work on pad systems has allowed AstroTurf to evolve through a series of developments. In the normal product development sequence for pad systems,

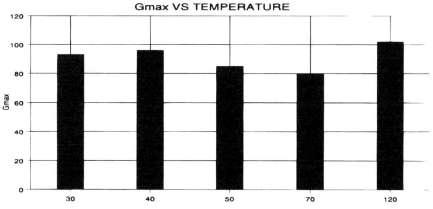

FIG. 2—G_{max} *versus temperature.*

APPENDIX

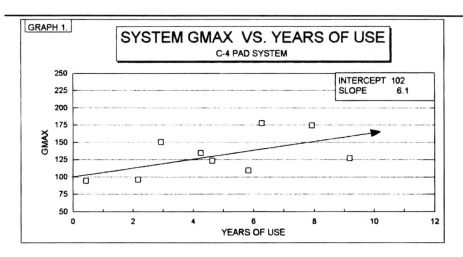

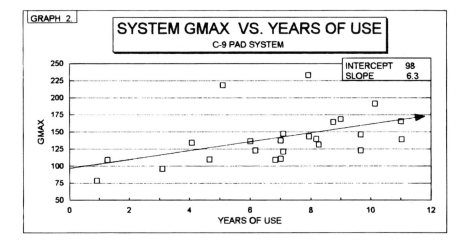

accelerated laboratory testing is used to predict beneficial changes or improvements. The true test is in extended field use. Periodic field inspections with impact testing are the best ways of analyzing actual performance.

AstroTurf developed many pad systems over the 30 years of synthetic turf usage. The pads and years of use are given below in Table 3.

Actual Turf/Pad System Performance in Field

Table 4 below shows the shift or increase in G_{max} values versus years of use, as obtained by linear regression of actual field G_{max} data collected over time (see Appendix). The reported values are means of G_{max} collected at predesignated playing areas on the field, in accordance with a standard grid test system. This standard grid sampling pattern called for testing a minimum of five (5) test sites per field with three impacts per test site. The G_{max} from each

APPENDIX

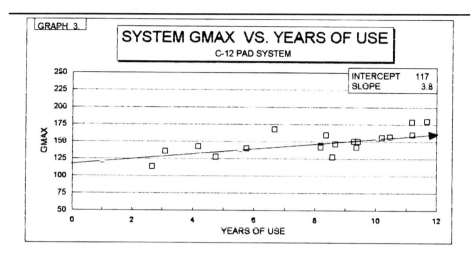

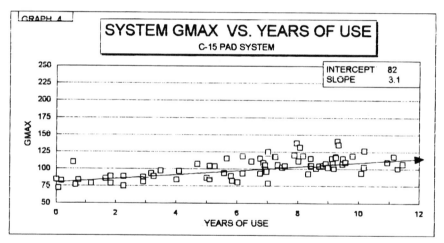

site was an average of the 2nd and 3rd drop, and the data reported in the Appendix are the mean average of the five (5) test sites or the mean value for each field impact tested.

The "intercept" values of Table 4 may be considered statistically-derived, initial levels of turf/pad G_{max} performance. The slopes measure at what rate G_{max} performance declines over the years. Because values of G_{max} up to about 150 continue to indicate good shock absorbence, it is apparent that fields remain serviceable for many years. Regular field monitoring is however essential to documentation of continuing good performance. The 200 G_{max} is considered the upper value for shock attenuation of American football fields according to ASTM Test Method for Shock-Absorbing Properties of Play Surface and Materials (F 355, Procedure A) both for natural and synthetic turf systems. Both type of fields have exceeded this value, and some older fields probably exist today that exceed this value.

APPENDIX

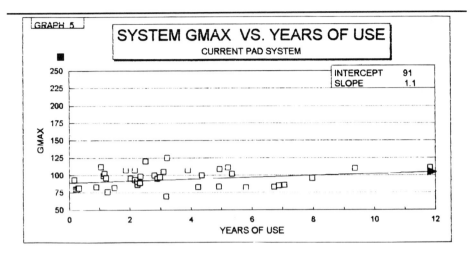

Summary and Conclusions

AstroTurf products have evolved with continued modifications and minor changes throughout the 30-year history of the product. The present product represents current optimization for player performance, product uniformity, playability, and longevity. New polymeric materials,

TABLE 3—*Major changes in Astroturf pad layer.*

Pad Code	Types	Years Used	Principal Improvement
C 4	Cross-linked pvc/nitrile rubber	1968–72	Good shock absorber
C 9	Cross-linked pvc/nitrile rubber	1972–80	Good shock absorbency combined with improved player comfort
C 12	Pvc plastisol	1972–78	Good comfort, somewhat higher G_{max}, improved G_{max} temperature response
C 15	Cross-linked pvc/nitrile rubber	1979–85	Major improvement in "C-9" formulation, higher density, improved physicals, improved adhesive bonding
C 25	Cross-linked pvc/nitrile rubber	1985-present	Fine tuning of C-15 series

TABLE 4—*Pad performance over time.*

Pad System	Standard Field Measurements	
	Intercept	Slope
C 4	102	6.1
C 9	98	6.3
C 12	117	3.8
C 15	82	3.1
Current	91	1.1

improved fiber spinning techniques, effective and environmentally friendly components, system design, and other technological advances will produce continual improvements in turf systems in future years.

Improvements in the materials used in field constructions and in installation techniques have improved the retention of the shock attenuation properties of latter generation of AstroTurf systems for American football. These latter generation field systems continue to indicate good shock absorbance retention properties compared to fields 30 years ago, although each individual field should be independently tested to measure its current shock attenuation properties.

Additional research and perhaps epidermological studies are needed to assess the "safety" of playing surfaces, both natural and synthetic turf, particularly lower extremity injuries that appear to relate to shoe-to-surface interface. The level of shock attenuations required for surface impact injury prevention may require additional research beyond the scope of this paper. Although, rule changes, improvement in protective equipment, and improvement in surface shock attenuation appear to reduce surface impact injuries, additional research is required to establish an upper limit of G_{max} for football fields.

References

[1] Orofino, T. A. and Hamner, W. F., *Encyclopedia of Polymer Science and Engineering*, Vol. 14, 2nd ed. 1988, John Wiley & Sons, Inc., New York, NY, pp. 245–260.
[2] Milner, E. M., Ed. *Comprehensive Guide to the World of Synthetic Turf*, Balsam Corporation, St. Louis, MO, (1993).
[3] Danforth, J. P. and Gadd, C. W., "Use of a Weighted Impulse Criterion for Estimating Injury Hazard," In Proceedings 10th Stapp Car Crash Conference, Society of Automotive Engineers, Detroit, MI, December 1966.

J. N. Rogers, III,[1] *J. C. Stier,*[1] *J. R. Crum,*[1] *T. M. Krick,*[1] *and J. T. Vanini*[1]

The Sports Turf Management Research Program at Michigan State University

REFERENCE: Rogers, J. N., III, Stier, J. C., Crum, J. R., Krick, T. M., and Vanini, J. T., **"The Sports Turf Management Research Program at Michigan State University,"** *Safety in American Football, ASTM STP 1305*, Earl F. Hoerner, Ed., American Society for Testing and Materials, 1996, pp. 132–144.

ABSTRACT: The turfgrass program at Michigan State University has recently dedicated and focused its research on sports turf management. There are three major areas of research: (1) the indoor turfgrass project, (2) the use of crumb rubber from used tires, and (3) management of high sand-based root zone athletic fields. The indoor turf project stemmed from the 1994 World Cup Soccer Matches involving the installation and maintenance of a portable turfgrass system in the Pontiac Silverdome in Pontiac, Michigan. The majority of the research for this project was completed in a 600-m^2 dome constructed on the Michigan State University campus specifically for this project. The crumb rubber project was initiated in 1990 and nine experiments were used to investigate the incorporation of crumb rubber from used tires into the soil profile and at the turf-soil interface of turf systems to improve turfgrass wear tolerance and reduce soil compaction. The sand-based root zone turf project was initiated in 1992 to investigate establishment and management scenarios specific to these areas. A 334-m^2 field was constructed to investigate these practices. Initial studies dealt with the establishment of either Kentucky bluegrass (*Poa pratensis* L.) or perennial ryegrass (*Lolium perenne* L.) with different fertilizer management regimes.

KEYWORDS: reduced light conditions, sand-based root zone, athletic fields, fertility, crumb rubber, impact absorption, traction, plant growth regulator, turfgrass

As a result of ever increasing use of sports fields and field safety issues, the sports turf manager faces a tremendous challenge to provide a high quality playing surface. Harper and coworkers [1] along with Rogers and Waddington [2] conducted studies demonstrating the relationship between agronomic practices and field conditions that ultimately affect player safety. Turfgrass science-related research has traditionally focused on golf turf, with information being subsequently transferred to the sports turf area. Because of the challenges unique to the sports turf manager (i.e., the inability to divert traffic and the intense use during suboptimal climatic conditions), there is a vital need for research specific to the problems of sports turf management.

Sports turf specific research in the United States has been limited [3]. Turfgrass research centers with these programs include the Pennsylvania State University, Texas A&M University, University of California-Riverside, and Michigan State University. The sports turf research program at Michigan State University has been in operation since 1989 at the Hancock Turfgrass Research Center. The research has centered around the following programs:

---

[1] Associate professor, research associate, associate professor, graduate teaching assistant and graduate research assistant, respectively, Michigan State University, East Lansing, MI 48824-1325.

- turfgrass management under reduced light conditions,
- crumb rubber from used tires in high traffic areas, and
- turfgrass management in high sand-based root zones.

The objective of this paper is to outline the major components of the sports turf research at Michigan State University. All of these projects have been designed to aid the sports turf manager in providing a high quality playing field with an emphasis on field safety.

Turfgrass Management Under Reduced Conditions

Many sports turf facilities have the option of using an artificial or a natural turfgrass surface. The exception to this option has been indoor facilities (i.e., domed stadia) that transmit insufficient sunlight to allow traditional turfgrass systems to grow and maintain adequate playing quality. Information regarding the maintenance of sports turf for indoor and other reduced light conditions before 1992 had been limited to the original construction of the Houston Astrodome in 1965 and a study conducted by Beard and coworkers [4,5] in 1991 at the Louisiana Superdome.

In 1991, the Pontiac Silverdome (Pontiac, Michigan) was selected as a site for the 1994 World Cup soccer matches. A mandate from the Federation Internationale de Futball (FIFA), the governing body for soccer, stipulated that all World Cup matches be played on natural grass. Officials from the Detroit Bid Committee and the Pontiac Silverdome asked for assistance from Michigan State University sports turf researchers to design, construct, install, and maintain a natural grass surface for the games inside the Pontiac Silverdome.

In August 1992, the Indoor Turfgrass Research Facility (ITRF) was constructed at Michigan State University. The ITRF was designed to emulate the environmental conditions inside the Pontiac Silverdome, thus allowing for the research and development of an indoor natural turfgrass field for the 1994 World Cup soccer games. The 600-m^2 ITRF was constructed using the same translucent, Sheerfill™ fiberglass fabric (Chemical Fabric Corporation, Buffalo, NY) used to cover the Pontiac Silverdome and other stadia and structures (e.g., Minneapolis Metrodome and the Denver International Airport). The fabric transmitted about 10% of normal sunlight (full summer sunlight is about 500-W m^2 of photosynthetically active radiation (PAR), the wavelengths of visible light between 400 to 700 nm required for plant growth). Generally, turfgrass requires at least 30% full sunlight (about 150-W m^2 PAR) for normal growth [6]. Reduced light conditions (RLC) occur at levels of light less than 30% sunlight. These conditions cause turfgrasses under traditional management programs to become weak, spindly, and eventually die from insufficient photosynthesis and intense disease pressure. Furthermore, shading from stadium structures blocks sunlight; therefore, most of the Pontiac Silverdome floor receives less than 5% of full sunlight. This level of light inside the ITRF was achieved by conducting the research during the winter months of 1992 through 1994 when the diminished natural solar radiation provided the equivalent of about 2 to 5% summer sunlight inside the ITRF.

The facility also simulated the Pontiac Silverdome in other respects. Positive pressure, supplied by built-in fans, supported the fabric covering the ITRF. Three 420-MJ furnaces were used to maintain the inside temperature at 16°C during the winter. In the summer, the facility was ventilated to maintain a temperature equal to that of the outside air temperature. Between the autumn of 1992 and the summer of 1994, testing was conducted inside the ITRF to develop a comprehensive installation and management program aimed at providing a portable turfgrass field for the 1993 U.S. Cup and 1994 World Cup soccer games held inside the Pontiac Silverdome. During this period, several tests were conducted under both ambient (2 to 5%

full sunlight) and supplemental (about 13% full sunlight) light regimes (Fig. 1). High pressure sodium lamps, 400-W each, were suspended 2.7 m above the turf to provide the supplemental lighting. Lighted plots were separated from unlighted plots by sheets of reflective mylar.

First in our series of tests, we evaluated the potential of multiple applications of the plant growth regulator flurprimidol, at several rates, to improve turfgrass quality under RLC. Under RLC, turfgrass plants grow weak and spindly as a result of an enhanced growth rate caused by excessive production of the plant hormone gibberellic acid (GA). Traffic rapidly reduces turf cover, resulting in a bare, hard surface. Flurprimidol has been successfully used on turfgrasses under natural light to reduce foliar growth [7] by inhibiting production of GA [8]. We evaluated flurprimidol rates on both Kentucky bluegrass and perennial ryegrass. In Test 2, the quality of Kentucky bluegrass was evaluated with and without flurprimidol at low, medium, and high nitrogen fertilizer rates (24, 49, and 98 kg ha^{-1} month^{-1}). Nitrogen rates were assessed because it is the major controlling element for turfgrass growth, and traditional management recommendations for turf in RLC recommend using only low rates [9]. However, the interaction of nitrogen with plant growth retardants on turfgrass under RLC had never been determined. In Test 3, Kentucky bluegrass quality, with and without flurprimidol, was evaluated over a six-month period under six light regimes: ambient light, 10- to 20-W m^{-2} PAR, 10- to 12-h photoperiod (ppd) (2 to 5% of the daily total of full summer sunlight); 40-W m^{-2}, 12-h ppd (13% of the daily total of full summer sunlight); 50-W m^{-2}, 24-h ppd (30% of the daily total of full summer sunlight); 75-W m^{-2}, 15-h ppd (30% of the daily total of full summer sunlight); 75-W m^{-2}, 24-h ppd (51% of the daily total of full summer sunlight); and 110-W m^{-2}, 24-h ppd (73% of the daily total of full summer sunlight). This test was designed to delimit the amount of light required for turfgrass to recover from simulated sports traffic. Our results agreed with Beard [6], showing that at least 30% simulated sunlight was required to maintain turfgrass of acceptable quality using traditional management techniques

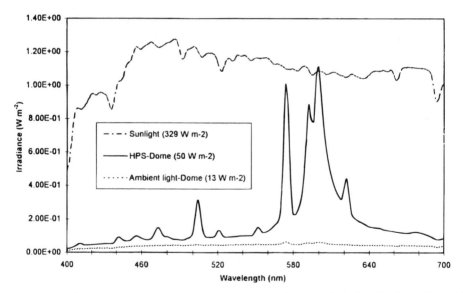

FIG. 1—*Solar irradiance transmitted through Sheerfill fabric into the Indoor Turfgrass Research Facility (ambient Light-dome), transmitted solar irradiance supplemented by 400-W high pressure sodium lamps (HPS-dome), and natural solar radiation outside on a sunny day. Data collected 10 March 1994, approximately 12:00 p.m., East Lansing, MI.*

(Table 1). Turfgrass died within four months at 2 to 5% sunlight, the ambient amount of light transmitted into the ITRF. At 13% simulated sunlight, turfgrass quality was reduced below an acceptable level. However, our other tests using nontraditional fertilizer and plant growth regulator (PGR) treatments have shown 13% simulated sunlight to be sufficient for maintaining high quality turfgrass under simulated sports traffic [10]. Applications of the PGR flurprimidol improved turfgrass quality and density at the lower light levels and improved turfgrass color across all light levels (Table 1). These results suggested that, with the use of a plant growth retardant, turfgrass quality can be maintained at a high level under RLC. Turfgrass density improved between 13 and 30% sunlight and was similar for all light levels tested over 30% sunlight. Turfgrass color was similar among the lower light levels within a PGR treatment, but declined dramatically at the two highest light levels, possibly as a result of chlorophyll degradation caused by constant illumination.

In addition to the above tests, a 30-m^2 portable "field" was installed inside the ITRF in January 1993 where it still stands today. The "field" was a prototype of the system used at the Pontiac Silverdome and consisted of ten steel hexagonal shaped modules (1.32-m length sides and 15-cm depth) with removable side walls. This component of the project helped to identify potential pitfalls in the system eventually used for the Pontiac Silverdome. Management of the "field" under the RLC of the ITRF has continued to provide critical information on the techniques required to maintain an indoor, natural grass sports field on a long-term or permanent basis.

In October 1994, the original Sheerfill fabric was replaced with a new version designed to transmit 16 ± 2% of natural sunlight. Research is continuing inside the ITRF to determine the potential for the long-term installation of turfgrass for sports stadia covered with the new Sheerfill fabric. Preliminary results with the new fabric show potential for the long-term installation of natural turfgrass athletic fields in covered stadia. We are convinced it is feasible to install natural turfgrass athletic fields for football, baseball, soccer, etc. inside covered

TABLE 1—*Color, density, and quality ratings for Kentucky bluegrass maintained under six light regimes in an indoor turfgrass research facility for seven months (December 1992 through July 1993).*

Light Treatment, W m^{-2}, Time	% Full Sunlight	19 July[a]					
		Color		Density		Quality	
		No PGR	PGR[b]	No PGR	PGR	No PGR	PGR
10, 10h	2.5	1.0[c]	1.0	1.0	1.0	1.0	1.0
40, 12h	13.0	5.0	8.5	2.7	4.0	1.8	4.0
50, 24h	31.0	5.7	6.8	6.2	7.5	5.3	5.3
75, 15h	30.0	5.0	7.0	4.7	6.7	4.3	6.0
75, 24h	51.0	3.0	4.0	6.7	6.5	5.7	5.0
110, 24h	73.0	2.0	3.7	7.0	5.8	5.7	4.7
	LSD (0.05)	1.0[d]		1.2		1.3	

[a]Rating scales are as follows: color: 1–9; 1 = brown turf, 9 = dark, uniform green color; density: 1–9; 1 = no living turf/bare ground, 9 = dense turf stand, no bare ground visible; quality: 1–9; 1 = brown turf/bare ground, 9 = dark green, dense, uniform turf stand. A rating of less than 5.0 is considered unacceptable.

[b]The plant growth regulator (PGR), flurprimidol (1.12-kg active ingredient per hectare), was applied on Dec. 18, 1992. 1 Feb. through 26 and 10 April 1993, according to label instructions.

[c]Turfgrass at this light level was nearly 100% necrotic by 10 April and completely necrotic by 17 May.

[d]Significant interactions ($p < 0.05$) were noted between light and PGR treatments for color, density, and quality ratings. Values are for means within columns and across rows.

stadiums for either short- or long-term usage. Further research is being conducted to define the appropriate management procedures for turfgrass under these and other types of reduced light situations.

Part of the research effort is devoted to evaluating cultivars of Kentucky bluegrass for their shade and traffic tolerance. Much of the current indoor turf research, however, is being conducted on a novel turfgrass species from Germany, *Poa supina* Schrad. Preliminary investigations by turfgrass breeders indicate *P. supina* possesses excellent shade, disease, and traffic tolerance [11,12]. *P. supina* has the unique attribute of a stoloniferous (aboveground lateral stems) growth habit which allows *P. supina* to recover rapidly in areas damaged by intensive sports-related traffic. No other cool season turfgrass used for athletic fields possesses this stoloniferous growth habit, thus athletic fields in the cool season areas are typically slow to recover from damage. A regular overseeding program is generally required to maintain even a semblance of turf cover on normal sports fields, but may not be necessary with a *P. supina*-based sports turf.

Crumb Rubber in High Trafficked Turf Areas

One advantage golf course superintendents have in combatting traffic on tees and putting greens is the ability to move or rotate tees and pins to distribute wear. In most cases, the sports turf manager does not have the ability to move high traffic areas. The consequence of this is the fierce battle to provide a turf cover in an area subjected to high traffic. This traffic causes excessive abrasion to the often young plant tissue as well as soil compaction, a condition not conducive to supporting turfgrass growth. To reduce susceptibility to compaction, high sand-content soils are used where high traffic is expected. Under these conditions, turfgrass wear or abrasion caused by both foot traffic and the quartz sand particle is difficult to avoid.

In 1991, it was estimated that 234 million tires were discarded in the United States with many of them in landfills. By 1994, because of public concerns, 25 states had prohibited these tires from landfills, and 46 states had legislated government funds to recycle the tires [13]. Research was initiated in 1990 through a set of experiments to address the environmental waste problem of used tires and develop a useful product referred to as crumb rubber, originating from used automobile tires. To manufacture crumb rubber, the tire must be stripped of the metal/steel and the fiber chords that reinforce the tire. From this point, the tire can be chipped into smaller pieces. It is these smaller pieces (6 mm or less) from which crumb rubber particles are derived. Such particles can be incorporated as a soil amendment into a variety of turfgrass situations.

The theory is that the crumb rubber particles introduced to the turf/soil environment system will increase turfgrass wear tolerance, reduce compaction, and subsequently reduce turf system inputs. Furthermore, it was hypothesized that with crumb rubber having elastomeric properties [14], it could provide a softer surface which could ultimately reduce the potential for surface-related injuries. Therefore, the objective of this research was to evaluate the feasibility and efficiency of incorporating crumb rubber into the soil profile or the soil turf interface in various amounts to measure turfgrass vigor and overall quality and playing surface characteristics.

The original and primary studies were initiated at our Michigan State University field facilities under a controlled situation. Crumb rubber (93% between 2.0 to 6.0 mm, 7% between 2.0 to 0.05 mm) was tilled into the soil to two final depths (7.6 and 15.2 cm) with five different volumes (0, 10, 20, 30, and 40% v/v). Total rubber incorporated at each depth was 0, 78, 157, 235, and 313 and 0, 156, 312, 468, and 624 t ha^{-1}, respectively. Perennial ryegrass (var. "Dandy") was seeded at 244.5 kg ha^{-1} on one plot, and another plot was sodded with Kentucky bluegrass. Before testing began, a three-to-four-month period of time was allowed for proper turfgrass development.

Field measurements for this study and all subsequent crumb rubber studies included impact absorption (Clegg Impact Soil Tester), traction (Eijkelkamp shearvane) [2], soil and surface temperatures (Barnant 115 thermometer), soil water content (gravimetric method), and soccer ball bounce. Laboratory tests included bulk density, adjusted bulk density as a result of the variation between crumb rubber particle density (1.2 g cm^{-3}) and soil particle density (2.65 g cm^{-3}), air porosity, and saturated hydraulic conductivity.

Traffic simulation was initiated with the Brinkman Traffic Simulator (BTS) [15]. Two passes with this device equal the amount of traffic received in one football game between the hashmarks between the 40 yardlines. On the average, three to four games were applied per week over a ten-to-twelve-week period for the duration of the experiment.

Impact absorption values and shear resistance are shown in Tables 2 and 3, respectively. There was minimal statistical significance as a result of tilling depths. On two of the three dates, as crumb rubber volumes increased, impact absorption and shear resistance values decreased on the perennial ryegrass treatment only. Because there must be a significant level of shear resistance maintained to sustain field quality as well as optimum impact absorption levels, it was determined that 20% (v/v) crumb rubber was the optimum amount to be tilled into the soil for this test.

Although these results were promising, it was difficult to introduce the crumb rubber into the soil. Therefore, the next step was to find the most efficient method of introducing crumb rubber to the soil/turf environment while still reducing compaction and increasing wear tolerance. Also, particle sizes less than 2- to 6-mm range needed to be evaluated.

In the next series of experiments, the two management practices used to introduce crumb rubber were core cultivation and topdressing. Both practices could expedite the process of introducing crumb rubber to the soil/turf environment while not taking a particular area or athletic field out of play. Because tilling depth was not significant in the previous study, both management practices allowed crumb rubber to be partially or fully above the soil surface. The area did not have to be stripped of the grass already existing and quarantined for re-establishment.

TABLE 2—*Effects of incorporation depths and crumb rubber volume rates on peak deceleration values on trafficked Kentucky bluegrass and perennial ryegrass turf, 1992.*

	Turf Species					
	Kentucky Bluegrass			Perennial Ryegrass		
Incorporation Depths, cm	26 Sept.	2 Oct.	20 Nov.	26 Sept.	2 Oct.	20 Nov.
	Peak Deceleration Values, G_{max}					
7.6	83	90	71	94	108	68
15.2	83	90	69	93	110	65
Significance[a]	NS	NS	NS	NS	NS	*
Crumb Rubber Volume, v/v						
0	92	97	73	96	116	70
0.10	87	97	75	96	112	70
0.20	79	84	69	96	109	67
0.30	79	87	70	93	106	63
0.40	80	86	65	89	100	62
LSD (0.05)	NS	9	7	NS	10	4

[a]Indicates a significant difference at 0.05 level.
[b]Indicates a significant difference at 0.05 level.

TABLE 3—*Effects of incorporation depths and crumb rubber volume rates on shear resistance values on trafficked Kentucky bluegrass and perennial ryegrass turf, 1992.*

	Turf Species					
	Kentucky Bluegrass			Perennial Ryegrass		
Incorporation Depths, cm	26 Sept.	2 Oct.	20 Nov.	26 Sept.	2 Oct.	20 Nov.
	Shear Resistance Values, kPa					
7.6	120	121	109	89	81	85
15.2	115	121	106	85	78	84
Significance	NS	NS	NS	NS	NS	NS
Crumb Rubber Volume, v/v						
0	116	118	103	100	91	91
0.10	115	128	107	99	85	87
0.20	115	121	107	91	81	86
0.30	122	121	111	72	76	82
0.40	120	118	110	73	67	76
LSD (0.05)	NS	NS	NS	16	10	5

The first study initiated in 1993 was the core cultivation experiment. The study was established at both the HTRC and the Michigan State University Marching Band practice field (MBpf), allowing evaluations to take place in both a controlled and uncontrolled environment. Furthermore, this procedure allowed for the evaluation of cleated traffic and regular foot traffic (sneakers and workboots; no cleats), respectively. The two particle sizes used were 2.0 to 6.0 and 2.0 to 0.84 mm (79.3% of particles between 2.0 to 0.25 mm and only 4.1% of particles between 0.25 to 0.05 mm). By using the previously derived appropriate rate (v/v) of 20% crumb rubber, a variety of cultivation treatments (Table 4) were implemented:

TABLE 4—*Effects of crumb rubber particle sizes and cultivation treatments on peak deceleration and shear resistance values at the Michigan State University Marching Band practice field, 1993.*

	Peak Deceleration Values, G_{max}			Shear Resistance Values, kPa		
Crumb Rubber Particle Sizes	21 Aug.	24 Sept.	18 Nov.	21 Aug.	24 Sept.	4 Nov.
2–6 mm	82	65	63	52	83	62
2.0/0.84 mm	82	63	63	59	80	67
Significance[a]	NS	NS	NS	*	NS	*
Cultivation treatments						
C5TD	80	64	61	51	77	60
C10TD	84	64	65	51	77	59
TR5	86	66	60	52	85	60
TR10	89	68	65	51	81	68
SSR	72	58	62	67	86	66
NOR	82	64	66	65	83	73
LSD (0.05)	8	4	4	7	NS	7

[a]Indicates a significant difference at 0.05 level.
*Indicates a significant difference at 0.05 level.

(1)   core cultivated five times + topdress crumb rubber + drag with mat to incorporate (C5TD),

(2)   core cultivated ten times + topdress crumb rubber + drag with mat to incorporate (C10TD),

(3)   topdress crumb rubber in between core cultivation five times + drag with mat to incorporate (TRS),

(4)   topdress crumb rubber in between core cultivation ten times + drag with mat to incorporate (TR10),

(5)   strip sod + till rubber 3 in. (7.6 cm) + resodded (1991–92 method) (TILL), and

(6)   check (cored five times; no rubber) (NORUB).

Traffic was applied by the Michigan State University Marching Band. Total size of the band ranged from 100 to 125 persons, and practice was conducted 4 to 5 times per week no matter the weather conditions. Footwear included sneakers and workboots: all flat-soled shoes.

Impact absorption and shear resistance results from the MBpf are presented in Table 4. These results were consistent with results recorded at the HTRC for 1993. For impact absorption values, there was a significant difference among crumb rubber treatments for all three testing dates. Shear values had a significant difference between particle sizes and among treatments for the same size on two out of three dates. At the beginning of the measurements, the trend favored the conventional tilling method and rubber treatments. However, as the season progressed all the treatments stabilized, and the crumb rubber treatments equilibrated to the forementioned treatments. Although data supported higher shearing values for the conventional and no rubber treatments in 1993, plugs of turfgrass appeared at the bottom of the shearing apparatus after the torque had been applied, indicating shallow rooting in these plots. Shallow rooted turf was observed sparingly with the crumb rubber treatments. This was consistent with the 1992 observations of shearing values in the previous studies. Although the turf had three or four months of turfgrass development, the sod had still not fully rooted. Even though the crumb rubber treatments were core cultivated, the turf plants had recovered and were ready for traffic. This translates to an athletic field potentially being ready for play in a quarter to half the time that the conventional method of incorporating crumb rubber to the soil/turf environment would require.

From previous observations, it was believed topdressing crumb rubber onto the turf/soil interface could provide benefits. However, only after an area had been fully reestablished and a 100% turfgrass stand existed was crumb rubber topdressed to the surface. If the study started from bare soil, there was the concern of crumb rubber absorbing too much heat as a result of its black color, thus adversely affecting new seedlings.

A topdressing study was initiated at the HTRC in 1993, and both particle sizes were implemented at five rates (0.0, 17.1, 34.2, 44.1, and 88.2 t ha^{-1}) into a mixture of 85% Kentucky bluegrass and 15% perennial ryegrass. The highest topdressing rate was determined based on 50% of the mowing height of 38 mm. The same field measurements were used to investigate playing surface characteristics [16]. In 1994, additional impact absorption character-istics recorded included total duration of impact (Tt), time-to-peak (Tp) deceleration, and rebound ratio (rr%).

Impact and other values for one date are shown in Table 5. (This table is a composite of the field measurements taken in evaluating playing surface characteristics. The numbers, under their respective categories were recorded following 92 passes with the BTS and were reflective of trends observed in 1994.) There was no significant difference between particle sizes for any of the measurements. Impact absorption, soil moisture, and surface temperature values were not significant among treatment values. However, Tt, Tp, rr%, and shear were significant among crumb rubber treatments. The latter four parameters were significant, with values

TABLE 5—*Effects of crumb rubber particle sizes and topdressing rates on a variety of field measurement values on a Kentucky bluegrass/perennial ryegrass stand after 48 football games simulated, 10 Nov. 1994.*

Crumb Rubber Particle Sizes	Peak Decel. G_{max}	Time of Duration Tt	Time to Peak Tp	Rebound Ratio rr%	Shear Resist., kPa	Soil Moist. %	Surface Temp. °C	Density %[a]
2–6 mm	60	10.3	5.7	0.22	63	16.3	8.6	60
2.0/0.84 mm	62	10.2	5.8	0.24	65	16.6	8.8	64
Significance	NS	NS	NS	NS	NS	NS	NS	NS
Crumb rubber Topdressing Rates, t * ha^{-1}								
0.0	58	10.1	5.6	0.17	52	16.2	8.7	42
17.1	60	9.1	6.1	0.18	67	16.5	8.7	51
34.3	62	9.9	5.5	0.21	60	16.8	8.7	63
44.1	61	10.6	5.7	0.26	70	16.8	8.7	66
88.2	62	11.1	5.8	0.31	68	16.4	8.8	88
LSD (0.05)	NS	1.0	0.4	0.03	9	NS	NS	14

[a]Density values recorded after 48 games simulated on 4 Dec. 1994.

directly proportional to crumb rubber rates. This translates to a softer, more resilient surface and an increase in traction on high trafficked areas, such as an athletic field. There was also an increase in turf density values as crumb rubber rates increased, thus showing the protection of the crown of the turfgrass plant by the crumb rubber.

From our original studies, crumb rubber revealed its ability as an ideal soil amendment in highly compacted areas. Also, we have found ways to introduce this soil amendment much quicker through core cultivation or topdressing or both. Furthermore, for athletic fields and high traffic areas, topdressing crumb rubber reduced surface hardness, improved turfgrass wear tolerance, and overall turfgrass quality and smoothness, thus reducing the potential of surface-related injuries.

Although crumb rubber is an excellent tool, it is not a "cure-all." Therefore, the use of crumb rubber cannot be an exclusive means for maintaining turf in any high traffic turfgrass area and must be used as a tool integrated into a management program.

Turfgrass Management in Sand-Based Root Zones

The challenge faced by the sports turf manager is to provide a high quality field under usually adverse conditions, often complicated by a high use period immediately following establishment. Sand-based root zones are gaining favor for athletic field construction since their soil structure does not change when exposed to frequent foot traffic [17]. One design currently being implemented with sand media is Prescription Athletic Turf, or PAT. The PAT system was developed at Purdue University under the direction of Dr. W. H. Daniel in response to the need for a safe and consistent playing athletic surface [18].

Despite the fact that there are over 25 PAT fields in operation as of 1994, there is little research information available regarding turfgrass management techniques in these sand-based root zones. The fields are built to use for contests, not research. In 1992, a 0.033-ha (330-m^2) PAT field was built at the HTRC with the intent to provide information regarding turfgrass establishment and management practices.

The management factors often questioned regarding sand-based root zones involve establishment techniques, field stability, and fertility regimes. For cool-season grass regions, Kentucky bluegrass and perennial ryegrass as monostands or in mixtures are accepted athletic field turf species because of their wear tolerance [19]. However, there is a lack of information regarding establishment procedures (i.e., sod versus seed) in sand-based root zones. When a sand-based athletic field's performance begins to fail it is often due to instability of the sand-based root zone. Irrigation and fertility can overcome most turf field problems, but will not improve soil stability [20]. In recent years, materials have been introduced in the soil profile with the intent of improving stability of sand-based athletic fields [21]. There is a need to evaluate the possibility of increased stability as a result of the inclusion of materials at the turf/soil interface. Proper fertility regimes for sand-based root zones are also unknown. Because sands have a low cation exchange capacity, they do not hold nutrients well and thus must be tested often to check for nutrient levels. The higher the sand content of the root zone, the more frequently fertilizers need to be applied. Because nitrogen is the major element controlling turfgrass growth, and the leaching or availability or both of nitrogen to the turf depends on the nitrogen form, information regarding turfgrass response in sand-based root zones to various nitrogen sources is needed.

The study was initiated at the HTRC in the fall of 1992. The experimental design was a 2 by 2 by 6 split-plot randomized complete block design replicated three times. Individual plots measured 1.5 by 3 m. The entire plot area was 0.0334 ha (334 m^2). The soil profile was 30 cm, 20 cm of sand (5.5% [2.0 to 1.0 mm], 38% [1.0 to 0.5 mm], 40% [0.5 to 0.25 mm], 10% [0.25 to 0.10 mm], and 1.5% [0.10 to 0.05 mm] by weight) only at the base of the root zone mix followed by 10 cm of the same sand mixed 80/20% with peat by volume. Two establishment methods were used, washed Kentucky bluegrass blend sod (KBG) versus a blend of perennial ryegrass seed (PRG). The second factor was a 4.0-cm-wide by 10.0-cm-long polypropylene fiber (known as VHAF, Notts Sports Ltd., Leincester, England) treatment included at rates of 0 and 1900 fibers m^{-2}. The third factor, split over the first two, was six fertility regimes: urea (46-0-0), IBDU (31-0-0), Lebanon (13-25-12), sulfur-coated urea, scu (32-0-0), Nutri-Plus (10-3-4), and Milorganite (6-2-0). On 26 Aug. 1992, Lebanon 13-25-12 was applied over the entire study area at a rate of 49 kg N ha^{-1}. Immediately before sodding or seeding, VHAF

TABLE 6—*The effect of establishment method, fiber inclusion, and fertility regime on turfgrass color, cover, and quality in a sand-based rootzone mix, 1993.*

Treatment	Color		Cover (0–100)	Quality	
	26 Oct.	23 Nov.	26 Oct.	26 Oct.	3 Nov.
Washed KBG sod	7.6	4.9	55	4.6	3.9
Per. rye seed	5.8	3.6	42	2.8	3.0
Significance[a]	a	a	a	a	a
Fiber	6.5	3.8	50	3.8	3.7
No fiber	6.9	4.5	47	3.6	3.1
Significance[a]	NS	NS	NS	NS	a
Urea (46-0-0)	7.0	4.6	46	3.7	3.3
IBDU (31-0-0)	6.1	3.8	50	3.5	4.0
Lebanon 13-25-12	7.5	4.9	56	4.7	4.2
SCU (32-0-0)	6.8	4.1	50	3.9	3.2
Nutri-Plus (10-3-4)	7.3	4.6	51	4.1	3.8
Milorganite (6-2-0)	5.4	3.1	39	2.5	2.3
LSD (0.05)	0.4	0.5	8	0.7	0.9
Games simulated	38	45	38	38	40

[a]Indicates significance at 0.05 level.
[a]Color scale: 1–9; 1 = brown, 9 = dark green, and 5 = acceptable.
[a]Quality scale: 1–9; 1 = bare ground, 9 = ideal turf, and 4 = acceptable.

TABLE 7—*The effect of establishment method, fiber inclusion, and fertility regime on turfgrass shear resistance in a sand based rootzone mix, 1993.*

	Date					
	10 Sept.	17 Sept.	24 Sept.	1 Oct.	11 Oct.	5 Nov.
Treatment	KPa					
Washed KBG sod	119	120	98	88	95	82
Per. rye seed	82	86	66	64	67	62
Significance[a]	a	a	a	a	a	a
Fiber	104	106	85	80	86	78
No fiber	96	100	79	72	77	67
Significance[a]	a	NS	NS	a	NS	a
Urea (46-0-0)	98	98	78	78	78	78
IBDU (32-0-0)	101	100	81	68	79	64
Lebanon 13-25-12	104	109	88	82	78	69
SCU (32-0-0)	102	107	83	78	93	73
Nutri-Plus (10-3-4)	102	105	84	78	81	80
Milorganite (6-2-0)	94	99	71	71	77	67
LSD (0.05)	NS	NS	NS	NS	NS	NS
Games simulated	10	14	18	23	28	40

[a]Indicates significant at 0.05 level.

fibers were laid down on the soil surface at a rate of approximately 1900 fibers m^{-2}. The washed Kentucky bluegrass sod was laid on 28 Aug. Perennial ryegrass was seeded on 29 Aug. at a rate of 245 kg seed ha^{-1}. The first fertilizer applications were administered at a rate of 24.5 kg N ha^{-1} for each respective fertilizer treatment on 19 Sept. The final fertilizer application for 1992 was on 9 Oct. at the 24.5-kg N ha^{-1} rate.

Biweekly fertilizer applications for all treatments resumed on 7 May 1993 at 24.5 kg N ha^{-1}. Monthly applications of 0-0-50 at a rate of 49-kg K_2O ha^{-1} were used to maintain acceptable soil potassium levels based on soil tests. At no time during the study was phosphorous at inadequate levels. Wear treatments were applied using the Brinkman Traffic Simulator beginning on 27 Aug. 1993, and the rate of traffic was eight passes per week, thus simulating four football games [*12*]. Traffic simulation was conducted Nov. 15 for a total of 45 games.

Data collected included turfgrass color, cover, and quality ratings along with root biomass and shear resistance. Analysis of variance was performed on all data, and means were separated using LSD procedures at the 0.05 level of probability.

Turfgrass color, cover, and quality data were taken during a high use period (i.e., Fall) relative to typical athletic field use and are presented in Table 6. Washed KBG sod had significantly higher color ratings compared to the PRG seed. No significant color differences were observed for the fiber factor. Significant color differences were noted for the fertilizer treatments. Complete fertilizer treatments (NPK) or quick release nitrogen sources had higher color ratings than slowly available nitrogen sources.

Turfgrass cover is the relative amount of surface area covered by turf. The washed KBG sod treatment provided significantly better cover by the end of the study than the PRG seed treatment. The fiber factor did not significantly affect turf cover. The fertility factor indicated that the Lebanon 13-25-12 treatment provided the highest cover, while IBDU and Milorganite resulted in the lowest cover. This is interesting because potassium and phosphorus levels were never shown as limiting throughout the study. The increased phosphorus and potassium provided by the Lebanon 13-25-12 treatment indicates the importance of each element during the establishment phase.

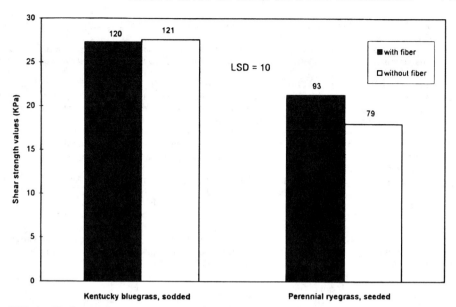

FIG. 2—*Turfgrass shear resistance as affected by establishment method and fiber addition, 17 Sept. 1993.*

Highest quality ratings were given to washed KBG sod. Quality of turf established from PRG seed was below acceptable levels late in the season as simulated traffic surmounted. The addition of fibers provided a significant increase in quality late in the season after 40 games of simulated traffic. Lebanon 13-25-12 provided the best quality ratings followed closely by Nutri-Plus, IBDU, SCU, and urea. Milorganite resulted in significantly lower quality ratings than the other fertilizer sources. No interactions for turfgrass cover or quality were observed for the dates provided.

Shear resistance measurements were taken after wear treatment was started in September 1993. Sod treatments had significantly higher shear values than seeded treatments through the study (Table 7). Fibers provided significantly higher shear values than treatments having no fibers. There was an establishment X fiber factors interaction on September 17 illustrating the benefit of VHAF fibers to the bunch-type perennial ryegrass seed establishment method (Fig. 2). No shear resistance differences were noted among the fertility treatments.

The establishment phase of athletic fields, especially sand-based root zone systems, is critical to their success. If established hastily and improperly, these fields will likely fail as a result of inadequate turf cover and poor and unsafe playing conditions. Sod establishment proved to be beneficial, as did the use of complete fertilizers as opposed to slow release or single nutrient carriers. Based upon this study, VHAF fibers placed at the soil surface before establishment were beneficial in limited evaluations and at no time were detrimental.

References

[1]   Harper, J. C., Morehouse, C. A., Waddington, D. V., and Buckley, W. E., "Turf Management, Athletic-Field Conditions, and Injuries in High School Football," Progress Report 384, Pennsylvania State University, College of Agriculture, Agriculture Experiment Station, University Park, PA, 1984.
[2]   Rogers, J. N., III, Waddington, D. V., and Harper, J. C., II, "Relationships Between Athletic-Field Hardness and Traction, Vegetation, Soil Properties, and Maintenance Practices," Progress Report

393, Pennsylvania State University, College of Agriculture, Agriculture Experiment Station, University Park, PA, 1988.

[3] Rogers, J. N., III and Waddington, D. V., "Present Status of Quantification of Sports Turf Surface Characteristics in North America," *International Turfgrass Society Research Journal* Vol. 7, 1993, pp. 231–236.

[4] Beard, J. B., "Indoor Turf," *Grounds Maintenance,* Vol. 27, No. 6, 1992, pp. 56–58.

[5] Beard, J. B., "Natural Turf for Domed Stadia-Feasibility Documented," in *Proceedings International Symposium on Soccer Field,* The Committee of International Symposium on Soccer Field and Soft Science, Inc. Japan, 1994, pp. 81–83 and 160–162.

[6] Beard J. B., *Turfgrass Science and Culture,* Prentice-Hall, Englewood Cliffs, NJ, 1973.

[7] Diesburg, K. L. and Christians, N. E., "Seasonal Application of Ethephon, Flurprimidol, Mefluidide, Paclobutrazol, and Amidochlor as They Affect Kentucky Bluegrass Shoot Morphogenesis," *Crop Science,* Vol. 29, 1989, pp. 841–847.

[8] Coolbaugh, R. C., Swanson, D. I., and West, C. A., "Comparative Effects of Ancymidol and Its Analogs on Growth of Peas and *Ent*-Kaurene Oxidation in Cell-Free Extracts of Immature *Marah macrocarpus* Endosperm," *Plant Physiology,* Vol. 69, 1982, pp. 701–711.

[9] Smith, T. M. and Rieke, P. E., "Lawns in Shade," Michigan Agriculture Experiment Station Bulletin E-1576, 110 Agriculture Hall, East Lansing, MI, 1986.

[10] Stier, J. C., Rogers, J. N., III, Crum, J. R., and Rieke, P. E., "Turfgrass Response to Nitrogen, Plant Growth Regulators, and Traffic Treatments in Reduced Light Situations," *Agronomy Abstracts,* American Society of Agronomy, Madison, WI, 1994, p. 185.

[11] Berner, P., "Entwicklung der Lagerrispe (*Poa Supina* Schrad) zum Rasengras," *Rasen-Turf-Gazon,* Vol. 15, No. 1, 1984, pp. 3–6.

[12] Lundell, D., "A New Turfgrass Species *Poa supina,*" *Grounds Maintenance,* Vol. 29, No. 6, 1994, pp. 26–27.

[13] Riggle, D., "Finding Markets for Scrap Tires," *Biocycle,* Vol. 35, No. 3, 1994, p. 41.

[14] Treloar, L. R. G., *The Physics of Rubber Elasticity,* Third Ed., Oxford University Press, 1975.

[15] Cockerham, S. T. and Brinkman, D. J., "A Simulator for Cleated Shoe Sports Traffic on Turfgrass Research Plots," *California Turfgrass Culture,* Vol. 39, Nos. 3 and 4, 1989, pp. 9–10.

[16] Rogers, J. N., III and Waddington, D. V., "Impact Absorption Characteristics on Turf and Soil Surfaces," *Agronomy Journal,* Vol. 84, 1992, pp. 203–209.

[17] Bingaman, D. E. and Kohnke, H., "Evaluating Sands For Athletic Turf," *Agronomy Journal,* Vol. 62, 1970, pp. 464–467.

[18] Daniel, W. H., "Prescription Athletic Turf System," in *Natural and Artificial Playing Fields: Characteristics and Safety Features, ASTM STP 1073,* R. C. Schmidt, E. F. Hoerner, E. M. Milner, and C. A. Morehouse, Eds., American Society for Testing and Materials, West Conshohochen, 1990, pp. 149–153.

[19] Cockerham, S. T., Gibeault, V. A., Van Dam, J., and Leonard, M. K., "Tolerance of Cool-Season Turfgrasses to Sports Traffic," in *Natural and Artificial Playing Fields: Characteristics and Safety Features, ASTM STP 1073,* R. C. Schmidt, E. F. Hoerner, E. M. Milner, and C. A. Morehouse, Eds., American Society for Testing and Materials, West Conshohochen, 1990, pp. 85–95.

[20] Gibbs, K. J., "Maintaining Surface Stability on Sand-Based Athletic Fields," *Grounds Maintenance,* Vol. 25, No. 3, 1990, pp. 58–64.

[21] Beard, J. B. and Sifers, S. I., "Feasibility Assessment of Randomly Oriented, Interlocking Mesh Element Matrices for Turfed Root Zones," in *Natural and Artificial Playing Fields: Characteristics and Safety Features, ASTM STP 1073,* R. C. Schmidt, E. F. Hoerner, E. M. Milner, and C. A. Morehouse, Eds., American Society for Testing and Materials, West Conshohochen, 1990, pp. 154–165.

Andrew S. McNitt,[1] *Donald V. Waddington,*[1] *and Robert O. Middour*[1]

Traction Measurement on Natural Turf

REFERENCE: McNitt, A. S., Waddington, D. V., and Middour, R. O., "**Traction Measurement on Natural Turf,**" *Safety in American Football, ASTM STP 1305,* Earl F. Hoerner, Ed., American Society for Testing and Materials, 1996, pp. 145–155.

ABSTRACT: An apparatus was developed and field tested to measure traction. The apparatus consists of a framework that supports a leg and foot assembly that can be used to measure both rotational and linear traction using different footwear under various loading weights. The force required to cause foot movement is measured at various degrees of rotation or linear distance traveled. Experiments were conducted to determine the effect of turfgrass and soil conditions on traction of turf areas. Specifically, the influences of species, cutting height, shoe type, and loading weight on traction were determined using this apparatus.

Tall fescue and Kentucky bluegrass provided the highest traction values while perennial ryegrass and creeping red fescue provided the lowest. Higher linear traction values occurred with lower cutting heights. As vertical force increased, traction increased. A studded shoe provided higher linear traction than a molded shoe across all species and cutting heights, while a molded shoe proved higher rotational traction under some conditions.

KEYWORDS: playing fields, traction, turfgrass, athletic footwear, cutting height, Kentucky bluegrass (*Poa pratensis* L.), perennial ryegrass (*Lolium perenne* L.), creeping red fescue (*Festuca rubra* L.), tall fescue (*Festuca arundinacea* Schreb.)

Athletic field playing surface quality can be defined as the suitability of a surface for a particular sport as measured (or perceived) in terms of the important interactions between the playing surface and the player or ball. An athlete interacts with a playing surface in two ways: through falling on the surface or through player to shoe to surface interactions. The effect the surface has on the surface-to-shoe interaction has been termed footing. Footing can be used to describe both smooth-soled and studded footwear. More specifically, the term "friction" has been applied to smooth-soled footwear and the term "traction" has been applied to footwear having studs, cleats, or spikes to provide extra grip. A playing surface should provide a level of traction that benefits the player's actions without causing excessive stress to joints or ligaments.

Canaway and Baker [1] have described a conceptual model of the factors affecting playing surface traction. These include the nature of the turfgrass, including its soil and plant constituents; external factors such as rainfall; management practices such as mowing and irrigation; and other factors such as pests and the amount of wear. The dynamic interactions between soil and turfgrass plants, with respect to traction, are not easily separated from one another.

Soil factors such as bulk density and particle size distribution may affect traction directly by influencing soil shear strength or indirectly through their effects on the turfgrass stand. More specifically, Canaway and Baker [1] stated it is how these soil factors affect water movement and retention and their interaction with wear that largely determine their effect on

[1] Research support associate, professor emeritus, and former graduate assistant, respectively, Pennsylvania State University, Department of Agronomy, 116 A.S.I. Building, University Park, PA 16802.

traction of athletic field surfaces. For example, it has been shown that traction on rootless soils increases with increasing soil bulk density [2]. However, on actual athletic fields, higher soil bulk densities are associated with the areas of greatest wear and have lower traction values due to a lack of turfgrass cover [3,4].

Studies of turfgrass plant factors, such as species, density, cutting height, and root mass, affecting playing surface traction have been reviewed [1,5,6,7]. Turfgrass and soil impart an influence on traction individually; however, traction on natural turf is often controlled by their combined effects.

Questions have been raised concerning the methods used to measure the horizontal forces associated with traction [8]. Differences among methods include shoe surface (sole type), vertical force applied, horizontal force applied (rotational or linear), and the value used to characterize the measurement (initial movement or peak value) [7]. The method that can best simulate the interaction of an athlete's foot in contact with the surface should provide the most meaningful measurement of traction.

In a review of the validity of methods used to evaluate the traction characteristics of a playing surface, Nigg [8] suggested that tests provide relevant information only when appropriate shoe soles are used and when the actual vertical force (loading weight) applied is similar to that applied by athletes. The review presents data from tests done to evaluate various artificial turf surfaces. The results demonstrated that by increasing the vertical force applied to the shoe-surface interface, the horizontal force needed to create linear movement of the shoe increased at varying rates for five artificial turf surfaces. One surface provided the least horizontal resistance of the surfaces tested at a vertical force of 280 Newtons (N) while providing the greatest resistance of the surfaces when tested at 770 N. Nigg [8] concluded that using vertical forces lower than those created by an actual athlete may lead to erroneous conclusions.

Middour [9] developed and tested an apparatus, termed PENNFOOT, that meets the requirements for valid traction evaluation set forth by Nigg [8]. This device has the advantage of measuring traction both rotationally and linearly, accommodating various athletic footwear, and using loading weights similar to those exerted by athletes. PENNFOOT is portable and measurements can be made *in situ*.

The objective of this study was to determine the effects of turfgrass species, cutting height, shoe type, and loading weight on linear and rotational traction. Traction was measured with the PENNFOOT apparatus in three experiments.

Procedures

Apparatus

PENNFOOT (Fig. 1), described in detail by Middour [9], consists of an inner- and an outer-frame. The inner-frame supports a centrally located collar through which a leg-shoe assembly slides. A set screw on the collar locks the leg-shoe assembly to the inner-frame during lifting or transporting. When the set screw is loosened the weighted leg-shoe assembly acts independently of the inner-frame. Wheels were mounted on the outer-frame for transporting.

The player leg is a steel rod with a ball-and-socket assembly on the upper end and a cast aluminum foot pinned on the lower end. The extreme top portion of the leg, above the ball-and-socket, is capable of being equipped with weights to exert various loading weights.

The simulated foot was cast from a size 10 foot mold. Two holes located on top of the foot are used for connection with the leg. The first hole located toward the toe allows the heel to be raised off the ground, distributing the weight on the ball of the foot. The second hole is used to place the entire sole in contact with the turf and distribute the weight evenly across the sole. All traction measurements in this study were taken in the toe stance with the heel of the foot raised off the ground.

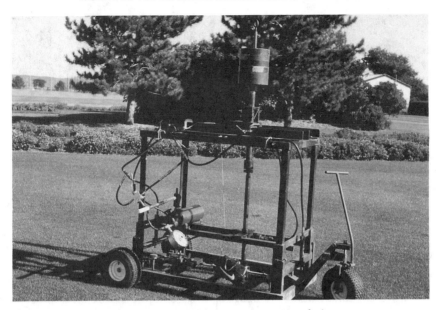

FIG. 1—*PENNFOOT traction measuring device.*

The horizontal forces associated with traction and the force required to lift or lower the internal frame were generated by a hydraulic hand pump. The rotating horizontal force was created by two pistons acting on a strike plate connected to the simulated leg. A protractor scale was used to determine how far the leg had rotated from the starting position. The linear force was created by using a single pulling piston that was mounted to the internal frame. The pulling rod was connected to the heel of the foot. The distance traveled by the foot was measured by a dial indicator. Raising or lowering the internal frame within the external frame was accomplished by two vertically mounted pistons. Prior to a measurement, the internal frame was lowered slowly by releasing the pressure, and the leg assembly was unlocked when the shoe contacted the turf. Thus, the foot was placed, not dropped, onto the surface.

A liquid-filled pressure gauge was connected directly to the pump to monitor the pressure being applied to the pistons. The pressure readings were converted to Newtons (N) and Newton meters (N · m) for linear and rotational measurements, respectively. Linear forces N were determined by calculating the product of the effective area of the pulling piston and the amount of pressure read from the gauge. Rotational forces were determined by calculating the moment of rotation. The moment of rotation is the force multiplied by the length of a lever arm, which for PENNFOOT is the piston strike plate.

Shoe Type

Two football shoes (Nike, Inc., 150 Ocean Dr., Greenland, NH) were used in this research (Fig. 2). The first shoe, referred to as the molded shoe, was a hightop with a molded sole that contained 18 triangular studs (12-mm long) around the perimeter of the sole and 35 smaller studs (9-mm long) in the center. The second shoe, referred to as the studded shoe, was a low-cut studded shoe that contained 12 cylindrical studs, each 12-mm long and 11-mm in diameter.

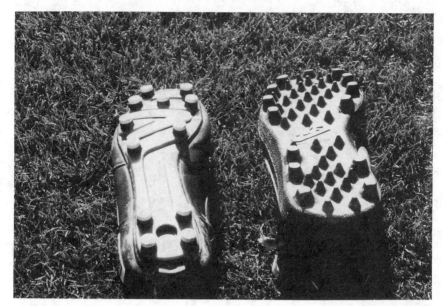

FIG. 2—*Studded and molded shoes used with PENNFOOT traction measuring device.*

Experiment 1

The effects of turfgrass species, cutting height, and shoe type were evaluated in this experiment. PENNFOOT was used to measure traction in June 1992, on plots located at the Joseph Valentine Turfgrass Research Center, University Park, PA. The soil type was Hagerstown silt loam (17% sand, 62% silt, and 21% clay). Four grass species, "Aspen" Kentucky bluegrass (*Poa pratensis* L.), Penn State 222 experimental perennial ryegrass (*Lolium perenne* L.), "Pennlawn" creeping red fescue (*Festuca rubra* L.), and "Arid" tall fescue (*Festuca arundinacea* Schreb.), were established in August 1990. The experimental design was a split plot (cutting height), split block (shoe type) design with three replications. Each species plot (5.49 by 6.10 m) was divided into three cutting heights subplots (1.83 by 6.10 m) for heights of 3.8, 5.1, and 6.4 cm. Blocks were split by shoe type (molded and studded). Linear traction measurements were made using a loading weight of 102 kg.

Experiment 2

In this experiment the effects of shoe type and loading weight were studied for both linear and rotational traction. Traction was measured on plots at the Landscape Management Research Center located at University Park, PA. This plot area was established in June 1990, with a mixture of three Kentucky bluegrass varieties (Fylking, Adelphi, and Touchdown). The soil was Hagerstown silt loam. The experimental design was a three-by-two factorial with three replications. There were three levels of loading weight (59.9, 88.0 and 116 kg) and two shoe types (molded shoe and studded shoe).

Experiment 3

This experiment was done to evaluate the effects of shoe type, loading weight, and soil water on traction on a high school athletic field constructed with a sand-modified soil. The experiment was conducted on September 10, 1992, on a football field at Preston High School in Kingswood, West Virginia. The turfgrass stand was a mix of Kentucky bluegrass and perennial ryegrass. The soil was a sandy loam (94% sand, 3% silt, 3% clay). Three areas along the length of the field were selected as replications. The areas were 5.2 m² and were located 2.3 m inside the hashmark. The areas were between the 10 and 15, 15 and 20, and 20 and 25 yard markers.

Experiment 3a—Using the studded shoe, rotational traction measurements were made on the plot areas with three PENNFOOT loading weight treatments: 59.9, 88.0, and 116 kg.

Experiment 3b—On the same plot areas used in Experiment 3a, rotational traction measurements were made using the molded shoe and a 116 kg loading weight. Results were compared with those obtained using the studded shoe in Experiment 3a.

Both Experiment 3a and 3b were repeated on three additional 5.2 m² plots located 2.3 m outside the same hashmarks so that results for inside and outside the hash marks could be compared.

Experiment 3c—After Experiment 3a and 3b data were collected, the field received a 2.4-cm rainfall during a 1-h period. Rotational traction measurements were then taken using a 116 kg loading weight and the molded shoe on both the inside and outside hashmark plots. These data were combined with traction measurements using the same loading weight and shoe type before rainfall in order to analyze the effect of soil water. The treatments will be referred to as pre- and post-precipitation.

Turfgrass Stand Characteristics

The turfgrass stand characteristics for the subplots in the experiments above were characterized using three 81 cm² by 2-cm deep plugs taken from each subplot in Experiments 1 and 2, and three 20 cm² by 2-cm deep plugs for Experiment 3. Above ground biomass and tiller density were determined using the procedure described by Lush [10]. The below-ground biomass was determined by first washing the soil from the roots and then determining the percent organic matter using Test Method for Moisture, Ash, and Organic Matter of Peat and Other Organic Soils (ASTM D 2974). Below-ground biomass was not determined for Experiment 3. Soil water content was determined by extracting four 2.4 cm² by 1.5-cm deep plugs from each subplot at the time traction measurements were being made for Experiments 1 and 2. Soil water content for Experiment 3 was determined using samples (7.65 by 2.0 by 5.0-cm deep) taken with a profile sampler.

Statistical Analysis

Four PENNFOOT traction measurements were used to characterize the traction of each subplot in the experiments. The mean values of the measurements were analyzed using analysis of variance. The least significant difference (lsd) at the 0.05 level was calculated when the F ratio was significant at the 0.05 level. For Experiments 3a, 3b, and 3c, the inside and outside hashmark data were then analyzed as combined experiments using the same level of significance just described.

Linear correlation coefficients were determined between traction values and the turfgrass stand characteristics in Experiments 1 and 3. Correlation coefficients were not calculated in Experiment 2 due to lack of degrees of freedom.

Results

Experiment 1

For all treatments in Experiment 1, traction values increased at a decreasing rate from 1.3 to 3.8 cm of linear travel and remained relatively level or decreased slightly from 3.8 to 5.1 cm.

Traction values among turfgrass species were significantly different at each increment of linear travel (Fig. 3). Tall fescue was significantly higher than perennial ryegrass and red fescue at linear distances of 1.9 through 5.1 cm of travel. Kentucky bluegrass was significantly higher than red fescue at all linear distances and higher than perennial ryegrass at 1.9 cm of travel.

The 3.8-cm cutting height treatment gave significantly higher traction values than those obtained from the 6.4-cm cutting height treatment between 1.9 and 4.4 cm of linear travel (Fig. 4). The results for both cutting height and species treatments are consistent with results reported in other studies [9,11].

The studded shoe yielded a traction value that averaged 140 N higher than the molded shoe. Due to experimental design, shoe differences were tested with an error term that had only two degrees of freedom. There were no significant differences due to shoe type; however, the species by shoe-type interaction was significant at 1.9 to 5.1 cm of linear travel (Table 1). Shoe differences were dependent on the grass species. For example, at 4.4 cm of linear travel, traction on Kentucky bluegrass using the studded shoe had a value 147 N higher than when using the molded shoe. Similarly, perennial ryegrass had a linear traction value 151 N higher with the studded shoe than with the molded shoe. Tall fescue had a much smaller (29 N) and insignificant difference in traction values between the two shoes. Red fescue showed the most dramatic difference with the studded shoe being 282 N higher than the molded shoe. These

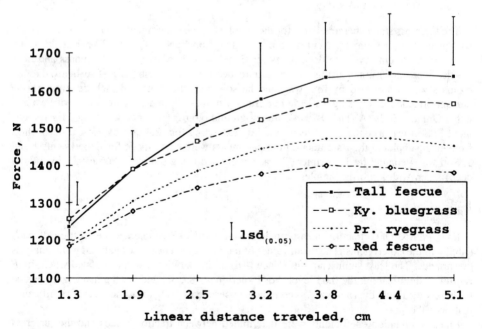

FIG. 3—*Mean linear forces for species across cutting heights and shoe type treatments for Experiment 1.*

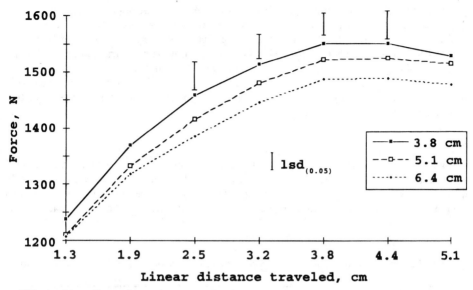

FIG. 4—*Mean linear forces for cutting heights across grass species and shoe type treatments for Experiment 4.*

TABLE 1—*Mean traction values for species by shoe type interaction obtained from Experiment 1.*

		Linear Traction, N						
		cm of travel						
Species	Shoe Type	1.3	1.9	2.5	3.2	3.8	4.4	5.1
Tall fescue	studded	1283	1405	1504	1576	1640	1659	1647
Tall fescue	molded	1191	1374	1480	1577	1632	1630	1628
Ky. bluegrass	studded	1339	1467	1541	1597	1643	1649	1634
Ky. bluegrass	molded	1174	1312	1387	1447	1502	1502	1490
Pr. ryegrass	studded	1298	1380	1447	1510	1535	1539	1527
Pr. ryegrass	molded	1088	1228	1321	1381	1409	1405	1376
Red fescue	studded	1269	1362	1449	1492	1535	1535	1529
Red fescue	molded	1100	1191	1230	1261	1265	1253	1230
lsd(0.05)		NS[a]	114	118	113	117	139	149

[a]NS = not significant at the 0.05 level.

relationships of a significant shoe effect with each species except tall fescue generally held true from 1.9 through 5.1 cm of travel.

One can also discuss this interaction according to the effect of the shoe on traction values obtained with the species. At no increment of travel were traction values significantly different between species when using the studded shoe; however, species differences occurred when the molded shoe was used. For example, a similarity in traction obtained with tall fescue and Kentucky bluegrass with the studded shoe occurred across the entire distance, but at 3.2 through 4.4 cm of travel with the molded shoe, traction was greater with the tall fescue.

Correlation coefficients between linear traction force at 3.8 cm of travel and soil water correlated positively for both the molded shoe ($r = 0.88$) and the studded shoe ($r = 0.62$)

across species. This correlation is probably due to an indirect correlation with species and not due to the effect of soil moisture on traction. Soil water contents between species were significantly different with tall fescue having the highest (0.21 kg kg^{-1}) and red fescue the lowest (0.14 kg kg^{-1}). There was no significant correlation between traction and soil water when examining individual species. Traction values obtained with the studded shoe were significantly correlated with below-ground vegetation ($r = 0.62$), while those obtained with the molded shoe were not ($r = 0.27$). There were no significant correlations between traction values and any other turfgrass stand characteristics measured.

Experiment 2

Significant differences for linear and rotational traction measurements are shown in Tables 2 and 3, respectively. Using linear measurements, the molded and studded shoes were significantly different at only 1.3 cm of linear travel; however, traction values were higher at each 10 degrees of rotation for the molded shoe as compared to the studded shoe when traction was measured rotationally.

TABLE 2—*Mean traction values for the designated variable obtained from linear measurements in Experiment 2.*

	Linear Traction, N						
	cm of travel						
Loading Weight	1.3	1.9	2.5	3.2	3.8	4.4	5.1
116 kg	1222	1414	1519	1607	1720	1752	1752
88 kg	1068	1179	1240	1348	1394	1417	1417
59.9 kg	867	949	998	1051	1071	1068	1068
lsd (0.05)	29	37	32	45	55	50	50
Shoe Type							
Molded shoe	1024	1170	1248	1331	1399	1416	1416
Studded shoe	1081	1191	1257	1339	1391	1409	1409
lsd (0.05)	23	NS[a]	NS	NS	NS	NS	NS

[a]NS = not significant at the 0.05 level.

TABLE 3—*Mean traction values for the designated variables obtained from rotational measurements in Experiment 2.*

	Rotational Traction, N · m			
	Degrees of Rotation			
Loading Weight	10	20	30	40
116 kg	22	28	33	35
88 kg	20	25	28	30
59.9 kg	15	19	21	22
lsd (0.05)	1	2	2	2
Shoe Type				
Molded shoe	20	26	30	32
Studded shoe	18	22	25	26
lsd (0.05)	1	1	2	2

Loading weights were significantly different at each increment of travel for both linear and rotational traction, with the heavier loading weights consistently yielding the higher traction values. There was no loading weight by shoe-type interaction.

Experiment 3

Traction values obtained with PENNFOOT for the main effects of the combined experiments are shown in Table 4. In Experiment 3a, loading weights significantly affected traction with higher traction values recorded for higher loading weights. Traction values inside the hashmark were significantly higher than those measured outside the hashmark only at 30 degrees of rotation. There was no experiment by loading weight interaction and no difference due to field location (replications) was found in Experiment 3a, 3b, or 3c.

In Experiment 3b, traction values obtained with the molded shoe were significantly higher than those obtained with the studded shoe at each 10 degree increment of rotation.

TABLE 4—*Mean rotational traction values for the designated variables for the combined experiments, inside and outside the hashmarks, for the main effects in Experiment 3a, 3b, and 3c.*

	Rotational Traction, N · m			
	Degrees of Rotation			
Loading Weight	10	20	30	40
	EXPERIMENT 3A			
116 kg	16.9	21.6	24.4	24.8
88 kg	14.8	18.5	20.8	21.1
59.9 kg	11.7	14.2	15.7	15.8
lsd (0.05)	0.7	1.0	1.1	1.2
Location				
Inside hash	14.7	18.4	20.8	21.0
Outside hash	14.2	17.8	19.8	20.2
lsd (0.05)	NS[a]	NS	0.9	NS
	EXPERIMENT 3B			
Shoe Type				
Molded shoe	23.2	30.3	33.5	34.1
Studded shoe	16.9	21.6	24.4	24.8
lsd (0.05)	1.4	1.5	2.1	2.4
Location				
Inside hash	20.0	25.8	29.4	29.6
Outside hash	20.1	26.1	28.6	29.4
lsd (0.05)	NS	NS	NS	NS
	EXPERIMENT 3C			
Soil water				
Pre-precipitation	23.2	30.3	33.5	34.1
Post-precipitation	20.4	26.8	30.8	31.0
lsd (0.05)	1.8	2.4	2.2	2.2
Location				
Inside hash	21.8	28.7	32.4	32.5
Outside hash	21.8	28.4	32.0	32.5
lsd (0.05)	NS	NS	NS	NS

[a]NS = not significant at the 0.05 level.

Pre-precipitation treatments, in which soil water averaged 0.13 kg kg^{-1}, measured higher in traction than post-precipitation treatments, which averaged 0.17 kg kg^{-1}, at each 10 degree increment of rotation in Experiment 3c.

No significant correlations existed between traction values and any of the plot characteristics measured.

Discussion and Conclusions

The results of each experiment have been summarized in the results section. This section examines trends or observations across experiments. The general shape of the response curves and the effects of loading weight, species, and cutting height are consistent with previous traction studies using PENNFOOT [9,11]; however, species effects on traction were confounded by shoe type and fewer significant differences were found than reported by Middour [9].

In Experiment 3, significantly lower traction was obtained on the sandy soil post-precipitation treatment using the molded shoe. Traction values did not correlate significantly with soil water values in Experiment 2 or 3. Soil water was not a treatment in Experiment 2, and as a result, the range of soil water values was small. In Experiment 1, there was no significant correlation between traction on individual species and soil water content. Traction with individual shoe types did significantly correlate with soil water content when considered across all treatments; however, this result was confounded by varying water contents across species. Traction values obtained with the studded shoe were significantly correlated with below-ground vegetation ($r = 0.62$), while those obtained with the molded shoe were not ($r = 0.27$). Because of the higher correlation of traction with the studded shoe, it is speculated that greater penetration into the turf occurred with this shoe. More research is needed on the effects of soil water on traction, and such research should include wider ranges of soil water contents on soils of various textures and having various amounts of turf cover. Stud penetration into the turf and soil should be addressed in such research.

Experiment 1 was designed to compare traction values obtained using the two shoe types across species and cutting heights. The studded shoe had consistently higher, but statistically insignificant, linear traction values than did the molded shoe when averaged across species and cutting heights. Traction differences due to shoe types were tested with an error term that had only 2 degrees of freedom. The magnitude of difference between peak traction values obtained with the different shoes was 148 N and is considered large when compared to other differences that have been found to be statistically different by this and other studies [9,11]. Significant shoe by species interaction did show shoe differences with three of the four turfgrass species. All linear traction values obtained on a species with the molded shoe were less than on the same species with the studded shoe, but this difference was not significant on the tall fescue stand. The reason tall fescue maintained higher traction values with the molded shoe was not apparent.

In Experiment 2, no differences in peak linear traction values were detected between shoes; however, in Experiments 2 and 3b rotational traction values obtained with the molded shoe were significantly higher than the studded shoe at each 10 degrees of rotation.

Under the conditions of these experiments, it can be concluded that when using PENNFOOT rotationally, the molded shoe yields higher traction values than the studded shoe. When using PENNFOOT linearly, a more complex picture emerged. In Experiment 1, traction with the studded shoe was consistently higher than with the molded shoe on three of the four species. In Experiment 2, however, there was little difference in traction values obtained with different shoes on Kentucky bluegrass.

Although all treatment effects were not consistent across all experiments, the results of these studies indicated that traction measured on natural turf can be affected by choice of horizontal force (linear or rotational), the loading weight, shoe type, turfgrass species, cutting height, and soil water content. In these studies, differences in shoe types were more apparent with rotational traction measurements. In other studies [9,11], traction differences due to varying turfgrass conditions including species and cutting heights were more apparent with linear traction. Before a standard method of measuring traction on natural turf is established, more work needs to be done to determine whether rotational or linear traction should be measured as well as a standard loading weight and shoe type. Considering interactions that occur, perhaps a standard traction test method should include more than one loading weight and shoe, as well as both rotational and linear measurements. Interactions among appropriate loading weights, shoe types, and surfaces are of importance to athletes and need to be addressed in future research.

References

[1]   Canaway, P. M. and Baker, S. W., "Soil and Turf Properties Governing Playing Quality," *International Turfgrass Society Research Journal,* Vol. 7, 1993, pp. 192–200.

[2]   Zebarth, B. J. and Sheard R. W., "Impact and Shear Resistance of Turfgrass Racing Surfaces for Thoroughbreds," *American Journal of Veterinarian Research,* Vol. 46, No. 4, 1985, pp. 778–784.

[3]   Rogers, J. N., III, Waddington, D. V., and Harper, J. C., II, "Relationships Between Athletic Field Hardness and Traction, Vegetation, Soil Properties, and Maintenance Practices," Progress Report 393, Pennsylvania State University, College of Agriculture, Agriculture Experiment Station, University Park, PA, Dec. 1988.

[4]   Gibbs, R. J., Adams W. A., and Baker S. W., "Factors Affecting the Surface Stability of a Sand Rootzone," *Proceedings of the Sixth International Turfgrass Research Conference,* Japanese Society of Turfgrass Science, Tokyo, Japan, 1989, pp. 189–191.

[5]   Bell, M. J., Baker S. W., and Canaway P. M., "Playing Quality of Sports Surfaces: A Review," *Journal of the Sports Turf Research Institute,* Vol. 61, 1985, pp. 26–45.

[6]   Canaway, P. M., "Playing Quality, Construction and Nutrition of Sports Turf," *Proceedings of the Fifth International Turfgrass Research Conference,* Institute National de la Recherche Agronomique, Avignon, France, 1985, pp. 45–56.

[7]   Baker, S. W. and Canaway, P. M., "Concepts of Playing Quality: Criteria and Measurement," *International Turfgrass Society Research Journal,* Vol. 7, 1993, pp. 172–181.

[8]   Nigg, B. M., "The Validity and Relevance of Tests Used for the Assessment of Sports Surfaces," *Medicine and Science in Sports and Exercise,* Vol. 22, 1990, pp. 131–139.

[9]   Middour, R. O., "Development and Evaluation of a Method to Measure Traction on Turfgrass Surfaces," M.S. Thesis, Pennsylvania State University, University Park, PA, 1992.

[10] Lush, W. M. and Franz, P. R., "Estimating Turf Biomass, Tiller Density, and Species Composition by Coring," *Agronomy Journal,* Vol. 83, 1991, pp. 800–803.

[11] McNitt, A. S., "Effects of Turfgrass and Soil Characteristics on Traction," M.S. Thesis, Pennsylvania State University, University Park, PA, 1994.

S. I. Sifers[1] and J. B Beard[2]

Enhancing Participant Safety in Natural Turfgrass Surfaces Including Use of Interlocking Mesh Element Matrices

REFERENCE: Sifers, S. I. and Beard, J. B, **"Enhancing Participant Safety in Natural Turfgrass Surfaces Including Use of Interlocking Mesh Element Matrices,"** *Safety in American Football, ASTM STP 1305,* Earl F. Hoerner, Ed., American Society for Testing and Materials, 1996, pp. 156–163.

ABSTRACT: Injuries on football fields can be grouped into different categories as related to the type of athlete movement and to the relative resiliency—softness of the surface. Many injuries are related to varying degrees of surface hardness. Turfgrasses offer the least hard surface in comparison to other alternatives available for sports activities. This is due to the biomass of the turf plus the associated root zone that provides a unique resilient characteristic or cushion.

Sports participant safety on turfgrasses is maximized by a dense biomass of turfgrass leaves and stems. It is important to select turfgrass species, cultivars, and cultural practices that have the capability of sustaining the highest possible biomass. Considerations in this regard include adaptation, wear tolerance, pest resistance, environmental stress tolerance, and the ability to recover from injury during the time of year when intense use occurs. Proper turf mowing, fertilization, irrigation, and cultivation practices also aid in maximizing the biomass cushion.

The second major dimension is the associated turfgrass root zone. High-sand/soil root zones of the proper particle size distribution are less prone to compaction and resultant hardness, plus the internal environment is more favorable for turfgrass root growth. The high-sand/soil root zones for sports use tend to be somewhat loose and thus benefit from stabilization, such as by the three dimensional, randomly oriented, interlocking 50 by 100 mm mesh elements. This mesh matrice also possesses a flexing action under traffic pressure that results in a self cultivation effect that further improves the environment for root growth by enhanced drainage and aeration.

KEYWORDS: football fields, turf, surface hardness, resiliency-softness, injuries, root zone, maintenance

Injuries on football fields and other sports surfaces can be grouped into different categories as related to the type of athletic movement and the relative softness of the turf-soil surface. Many impact-type injuries are related to varying degrees of surface hardness, with the safety of the participant increasing inversely with a lessening of surface hardness. There are other surface playability characteristics of concern, such as traction, wear tolerance, divot opening/ turf recovery, and smoothness. This paper will primarily address the aspect of hardness of natural surfaces.

[1]Turfgrass research associate, Turfgrass Physiology, Texas A&M University; now, associate agronomist, International Sports Turf Institute, 2204 Bristol, Bryan, TX 77802.

[2]Professor Emeritus of Turfgrass Science, Texas A&M University; now, President of International Sports Turf Institute, 1812 Shadowood Dr., College Station, TX 77840.

Surface Hardness Assessment

The hardness and resultant safety of a surface can be measured using a lightweight portable apparatus, the Clegg Impact Soil Tester. Several models of this device, with differing hammer weights of 0.5, 2.25, and 4.5 kg, are used in turf research. Each provides a relative scale of impact resistance of the surface measured in gravities (g), with a decreasing number indicating a lessening of hardness.

Comparisons of surface hardness for a variety of surfaces, from concrete to turfed soil, as assessed by the Clegg device with a hammer weight of 2.25 kg, are shown in Table 1. Results indicate a decrease in surface hardness as the composition of the material becomes less dense. Major differences in hardness occur among solids: (a) materials such as cement, composition, or wood floor surfaces; (b) other types of artificial playing surfaces; and (c) the natural turf-soil surfaces. Turfgrasses offer the least hard surface in comparison to other alternatives available for sports activities. This is due to the biomass of the turf and the associated root zone that provide a uniquely resilient characteristic and cushion. Differences occur within the natural turf-soil surfaces with changes in: (a) soil texture, (b) moisture content, and (c) whether the surface is bare soil or turfed.

Turfgrass Effects

Sports participant safety on natural turfgrass is maximized through providing a dense biomass of above ground turfgrass leaves, shoots, and stems grown on a stable, low-density root zone. It therefore is important to select the correct turfgrass species/cultivar, root zone, and cultural practices that have the capability of sustaining the highest possible biomass over the entire use period. Considerations should include the turfgrass species/cultivar adaptation, turfgrass wear tolerance, pest resistance, environmental stress tolerance, and the ability to recover rapidly from turf injury during the time of year when intense use occurs. Proper turfgrass fertilization, irrigation, and cultivation practices also aid in maximizing the biomass cushion, thus lessening surface hardness. Results of several of our cultural studies as described in the following paragraphs illustrate these effects.

Cutting Height Effects

Surface hardness of turfed sport venues can be modified by changing the height of cut. This was shown in our study with Tifway bermudagrass (*Cynodon dactylon* x *C. transvaalensis*)

TABLE 1—*Comparisons of the hardness of representative surfaces in the College Station, Texas area expressed as means of multiple observations of Clegg Impact Value (CIV) using the 2.25-kg hammer weight with the fourth drop reading from a 300-mm height.*

Representative Surface Types	Clegg Impact Value, g
	2.25-kg Hammer
Cement floor	1426
Asphalt road	1442
Tennis court—outdoor composition	1422
Composition running track	1432
Basketball court—permanent wood	640
Football stadium—outdoor, 4-year-old artificial surface	175
Football stadium—indoor, 1-year-old artificial surface	141
Baseball—bare clay infield	504
Baseball—natural turfed field of bermudagrass	100

grown on a modified high-sand root zone at seven heights of cut from 12 to 250 mm. Total shoot biomass density was determined by counting the shoots per square decimetres harvesting and obtaining dry weight of shoots per square decimetres. As the height of cut increased the number of shoots per square decimetres decreased at each of the seven heights. The dry weight of the shoots per square decimetres decreased at each height up to 100 mm then increased at 250 mm. This was accompanied by a decrease in surface hardness from 12 to 25 mm, then a stable reading to 50 mm and another plateau to 100 mm followed by a further decrease to 250 mm (Table 2). All results were within the acceptable range specified in the standard for surface playability of football (soccer) fields (10 to 100 g) proposed by the Sports Turf Research Institute, United Kingdom, and the acceptable running range in the proposed standard for turfed horse racing surfaces (30 to 110 g) of the authors [1]. Although we assessed seven heights of cut in our study, the most appropriate turfgrass cutting height for football and other field sports from playability and turfgrass health viewpoints ranges from 12 to 50 mm. Turfed horse racing surfaces generally have cutting heights of 100 mm.

Nitrogen Fertility Effects

Smaller changes in surface hardness can be made by increasing the nitrogen fertility rate within the same height of cut (Table 3). The increased nitrogen fertility resulted in increased shoot biomass at each of three heights. However, in this study, the height of cut effect on surface hardness was more dominate than the effect of an increased nitrogen nutritional level.

Turfgrass Cultivar Effects

The effects of *Zoysia* cultivar selection and two heights of cut using the 0.5-kg hammer and the fourth drop indicate that surface hardness can be modified by cultivar selection and by height of cut. The softness benefits exceeded 50% among these six cultivars (Table 4). The increasing softness among cultivars was associated with an increase in shoot density and a higher leaf to stem ratio. The effects of an increased cutting height on enhanced softness of the surface were substantial as reported earlier.

Root Zone Effects

Aside from turfgrass species/cultivar selection and culture, the other primary component that can be modified to decrease the hardness of natural turfgrass surfaces is via selection of

TABLE 2—*Effects of seven heights of cut on surface hardness expressed as five-year means of the Clegg Impact Value (CIV) (fourth drop) for mature Tifway bermudagrass* (Cynodon dactylon x C. transvaalensis) *grown on a modified high-sand root zone, 1989 to 1994.*

	Clegg Impact Value, g
Height of Cut, mm	2.25-kg Hammer
12	62 a*
25	58 bc
37	57 c
50	54 cd
75	51 d
100	51 d
250	47 e

*Means followed by the same letter within the same column are not significantly different at the 5% level, LSD *t*-test.

TABLE 3—*Effects of three heights of cut and three nitrogen (N) fertilization levels on surface hardness expressed as five-year means on the Clegg Impact Value (CIV) (fourth drop) for mature Tifway bermudagrass* (Cynodon dactylon x C. transvaalensis) *grown on a modified high-sand root zone, 1989 to 1994.*

Height of Cut, mm	Nitrogen Rate Per Growing Month, N kg/100 m^2	Clegg Impact Value, g 2.25-kg Hammer
12	0.25	62 a*
12	0.50	58 ab
12	0.75	53 b
25	0.25	58 ab
25	0.50	53 b
25	0.75	60 ab
37	0.25	60 ab
37	0.50	59 ab
37	0.75	55 b

*Means followed by the same letter within the same column are not significantly different at the 5% level, LSD *t*-test.

TABLE 4—*Effects of six mature* Zoysia *cultivar turfs and two heights of cut on the surface hardness expressed as the Clegg Impact Value (CIV) using a 0.5-kg hammer weight and the fourth drop from a 300-mm height. Root zone is a modified high-sand.*

Zoysia Grass	Height of Cut, mm		% Change from 12- to 25-mm Cutting Heights
	12 mm	25 mm	
Belair	69 a*	41 a	−41
El Toro	54 b	39 a	−28
Korean Common	55 b	35 a	−36
Meyer	48 bc	33 a	−31
FC 13251	44 c	31 ab	−30
Emerald	32 d	22 b	−31

*Means followed by the same letter within the same column are not significantly different at the 5% level, LSD *t*-test.

the associated turfgrass root zone. Assessments shown in Table 5 indicate an increase in surface hardness occurred with changes in soil texture from high sand to soils having more silt and clay. The range in CIV for the 2.25-kg hammer weight on bare soils was 91 to 132 g and for turfed soils 88 to 116 g. There was 3 to 16% less hardness in turfed surfaces versus bare soil. The CIV's for the three soils were within the acceptable range of the two proposed standards. Soils with a high clay content develop, over time, a serious compaction problem that increases hardness and results in a very unfavorable environment for root growth of turfgrasses.

The ever increasing intensity of traffic on golf greens, sports fields, and horse race tracks during the past three decades necessitated the development and use of high-sand root zones, such as the Texas-USGA Method [2], for construction of root zones. This development minimized serious soil compaction problems and provided a higher quality, safer turfed playing surface. However, these root zones were relatively unstable under certain playing conditions.

TABLE 5—*Comparisons of the hardness of four moist nonturfed and Tifway bermudagrass (Cynodon dactylon x C. transvaalensis) turfed root zones expressed as means of multiple observations over three years of the Clegg Impact Value (CIV) using the 2.25-kg hammer weight and the fourth drop reading from a 300-mm height.*

| | Clegg Impact Value, g | | |
| | 2.25-kg Hammer | | |
Root Zone Texture	Soil Only	Soil and Turf	% Change
High-sand mix (95% sand, 2% silt, 3% clay)	91	88	−3
Sandy loam (86% sand, 6% silt, 8% clay)	102	97	−5
Sandy clay loam (65% sand, 12% silt, 23% clay)	120	107	−13
Clay loam (47% sand, 24% silt, 29% clay)	132	116	−16

Mesh Inclusion Effects

In 1985, the authors began a series of long-term investigations at Texas A&M University to assess the use of randomly oriented, interlocking mesh elements for stabilization of high-sand root zones, while also enhancing the environment for turfgrass root growth. These investigations were subsequently expanded in 1990 to include root zones with sandy clay loam and clay loam soil textures.

The mesh elements, manufactured by Netlon Ltd., consist of discrete 50- to 100-mm rectangular units that have dimensional stability and flexural stiffness. Each element has open ribs extending from the perimeter and a square aperture between the mesh ribs of 10 by 10 mm. The open ribs facilitate an interlocking structure that provides a unique three-dimensional (3-D) matrix of a relatively fixed, but microflexible, nature. This three-dimensional, interlocking mesh element-root zone is distinctly different from the two-dimensional, noninterlocking, nonstabilized, fibrillated polypropolene fibers.

The mesh elements were combined with the soils in specific amounts of 2.5, 3.75, or 5.0 kg/m^3 of soil, with rigorous mixing to ensure a completely random orientation of the mesh element pieces. The mesh-soil mix was then installed to a depth of 150 mm over a 150-mm depth of the same soil without mesh elements that had been placed over a prepared subbase that included a drainage system. Three replicate plots of each mesh density rate and three plots of the same soil without mesh elements were then compared. In most of the studies, a topdressing with 25 mm of the same soil without mesh elements was placed over the mesh/soil matrix before planting the turfgrass, while one replication was not topdressed. This top layer proved to be of significant benefit, especially in the divot size and divot opening turf recovery assessments.

Two traffic stress components were assessed over a four-year period. The turf wear components were characterized by the divot opening length, width, and depth; the rate of turf recovery in the divot openings; and the turf tear. The second traffic stress component, soil compaction, also was assessed via water infiltration rate, percolation rate, and surface hardness. Playing surface characteristics assessed were traction, ball bounce, surface hardness, and compressive displacement. Soil moisture retention and turfgrass quality also were determined.

Results of the original field assessments were summarized in an earlier ASTM publication [1]. Results of the subsequent field studies conducted at Texas A&M University, which have been conducted for a minimum of three years for each soil texture, are remarkably similar, except for scale. Generally, as the volume of the interlocking mesh elements added to the root zone increased, there was a corresponding enhancement of the root zone/turfgrass complex, regardless of the soil texture, with the 5.0-kg inclusion rate being best. There were relative scale differences between soils of different texture in some of the assessments. However, in all cases, the addition of interlocking mesh elements was beneficial when compared to the same soil without mesh elements.

Surface hardness results shown in Table 6 indicate that, with the 2.25 kg-hammer, the range of CIVs for turfed soils with interlocking mesh elements was 69 to 87 g or 19 to 29% less hard than the same turfed soils without mesh. All of the soils containing interlocking mesh elements were within the acceptable playability range. The mesh imparted a dramatic improvement in relative softness of the surface providing a cushion against potential injuries to sports participants.

Results of three other assessments affecting turfed natural surface sport fields are included in this report: divot size, divot opening turf recovery, and water infiltration rate. Assessment apparatus used for these studies are described in the earlier referenced ASTM publication [1] or in Ref [2]. Divot size assessments for no mesh and interlocking mesh element inclusions in three turfed soil textures are compared in Table 7. Divot opening lengths were decreased by the addition of interlocking mesh elements in all three soils, with the improvement ranging from 24 to 49%. Divot opening width also was improved by 14 to 22% as a result of interlocking mesh inclusion.

The turf recovery of these divot openings for root zones with interlocking mesh inclusions was from 29 to 41% more rapid when expressed as days to 50% turf recovered, and 29 to 37% more rapid at the 75% turf recovery point (Table 8). The clay loam soil was the slowest in turf recovery, requiring 25 and 30 days, respectively.

The water infiltration rates, assessed with a double ring infiltrometer, were highest for the sand root zones and lowest for the clay loam root zones, but within each soil type an improvement was

TABLE 6—*Effects of interlocking mesh elements on the hardness of four moist Tifway bermudagrass* (Cynodon dactylon x C. transvaalensis) *turfed root zones expressed as means of multiple observations over three years of the Clegg Impact Value (CIV) using the 2.25-kg hammer weight with the fourth drop reading from a 300-mm height.*

| | Clegg Impact Value, ,g 2.25-kg Hammer | | |
Root Zone Texture	No Mesh	Mesh	% Change
High sand	88	69	−19
Sandy loam	97	76	−19
Sandy clay loam	107	84	−23
Clay loam	116	87	−29

TABLE 7—*Comparisons of divot opening length and divot opening width for mature Tifway bermudagrass* (Cynodon dactylon x C. transvaalensis) *grown on three distinct root zones modified by 5.0 kg m^{-3} of interlocking mesh element inclusions versus not modified.*

| | Divot Opening Length, mm | | | Divot Opening Width, mm | | |
Root Zone Texture	No Mesh	Mesh	% Change	No Mesh	Mesh	% Change
Sand	134*	102*	−24	55*	46*	−16
Sandy clay loam	141	95	−33	49	42	−14
Clay loam	149	76	−49	54	42	−22

*Means of four individual assessments per year over three years.

TABLE 8—*Comparisons of divot opening turf recovery time for mature Tifway bermudagrass* (Cynodon dactylon x C. transvaalensis) *grown on three distinct root zones modified with 5.0 kg m^{-3} of interlocking mesh element inclusions versus not modified.*

Root Zone Texture	Divot Opening Turf Recovery					
	Days to 50% Recovery			Days to 75% Recovery		
	No Mesh	Mesh	% Change	No Mesh	Mesh	% Change
Sand	21*	14*	−33	28*	20*	−29
Sandy clay loam	32	19	−41	41	26	−37
Clay loam	35	25	−29	46	30	−35

*Means of four individual assessments per year over three years.

TABLE 9—*Comparisons of water infiltration into mature Tifway bermudagrass* (Cynodon dactylon x C. transvaalensis) *turf-root zones modified by 5.0-kg m^{-3} interlocking mesh element inclusions versus not modified.*

Root Zone Texture	Infiltration Rate, mm/h		
	No Mesh	Mesh	% Change
Sand	571*	1069*	+47
Sandy clay loam	<10	113	+91
Clay loam	<5	75	+93

*Means of four individual assessments per year over three years.

noted as a result of interlocking mesh element inclusion in the root zone (Table 9). The improvement varied from 47% for a sand to 93% for a clay loam root zone.

Summary

These studies indicate that surface hardness can be decreased, with resultant increases in participant safety, through selection of turfgrass species/cultivar, height of cut, nitrogen fertility regime, root zoil texture, and use of interlocking mesh element inclusions.

Based on these and other studies by the author, the benefits that are to be expected from the addition of interlocking mesh elements to a turfed installation with a root zone of any soil texture are the following:

- enhanced soil stabilization,
- less surface hardness,
- enhanced participant safety,
- improved load-bearing capacity,
- resistance to surface rutting,
- 24 to 49% reduction in divot size,
- 29 to 41% faster divot opening turf recovery,
- improved uniformity of ball bounce,
- decreased soil compaction,
- comparable traction,

- internal microflexing for aeration,
- increased water infiltration and percolation,
- improved soil moisture retention, and
- improved turfgrass rooting and overall turf health.

Although these benefits are realized within each soil type and each volume of interlocking mesh inclusion, the best overall root zone in these assessments was the high-sand root zone with a 5.0-kg/m^3 volume of interlocking mesh elements and an inclusion depth of 150 mm.

Potential uses for this interlocking mesh elements/turfgrass root zone complex are numerous. Major installation types now in existence using the mesh are sports fields, golf course tees and cart paths, turfed horse race tracks, equestrian event arenas and show grounds, turfed roadways and parking areas, and other heavy load-bearing areas such as fire truck access lanes.

To achieve this type of multifunctional surface that performs under a range of diverse stresses, it will be somewhat more expensive to install. However, it will function for a longer time and accommodate a much larger number of events, recreational activities, or traffic pressures, which, in the long term, makes this system far more cost-effective. Additionally, this system may provide the only answer to some unique, severe-stress turfgrass problems that had no solution in the past.

References

[1]   Beard, J. B and Sifers, S. I., "Feasibility Assessment of Randomly Oriented Interlocking Mesh Element Matrices for Turfed Root Zones," *ASTM STP 1073, Natural and Artificial Playing Fields: Characteristics and Safety Features,* American Society for Testing and Materials, West Consho-hocken, PA, 1990, pp. 154–165.

[2]   Beard, J. B and Sifers, S. I., "Stabilization and Enhancement of Sand-Modified Root Zones for High Traffic Sports Turfs with Mesh Elements," Texas Agricultural Experiment Station, Texas A&M University System, B-1710, 1993, 40 pp.

[3]   Beard, J. B and Sifers, S. I., "A Randomly Oriented, Interlocking Mesh Element Matrices System for Sport Turf Root Zone Construction," in *Proceedings of the International Turfgrass Research Conference,* Vol. 6, 1989, pp. 253–257.

[4]   Sifers, S. I., Beard, J. B, and Hall, M. H., "Turf Plant Responses and Soil Characterizations in Sandy Clay Loam and Clay Loam Soil Augmented by Turf in Interlocking Mesh Elements—1992," Texas Turfgrass Research, Texas Agricultural Experiment Station, College Station, TX, PR-5142, 1993, pp. 112–116.

Management: Systems

Richard P. Borkowski[1]

The Football Coach and Football Safety

REFERENCE: Borkowski, R. P., "**The Football Coach and Football Safety,**" *Safety in American Football, ASTM STP1305,* Earl F. Hoerner, Ed., American Society for Testing and Materials, 1996, pp. 167–171.

ABSTRACT: The game of football and especially those that play it, have benefitted from the extensive improvements that lower the potential for injuries. Equipment, facilities, and the general body of sports medicine knowledge have all helped to lower the chances of minor and major injuries.

The most important factor for safety in American football, however, has been and continues to be the attitude and skill of the coach.

This paper addresses those attitudes and skills that a coach must possess to offer a worthwhile and safe experience to those in his charge. This paper addresses the human factor in football safety. It further offers a list of situations to avoid within the football atmosphere that are based on this author's personal litigation experience. This paper makes several proposals to improve the safety quotient in football.

KEYWORDS: warn, supervise, equipment, facilities, conditioning, post care, instruction, coach, avoid, tackle, associations, expert witness

The safety advancements in the game of American football have been extensive during recent decades. Improvements in equipment, facilities, rules, conditioning requirements, and sports medicine must continue to lower the probability of injury in this exciting yet high risk sport [1].

My 34-year experience as a school coach and athletic administrator, as well as being what society calls an "expert witness," strongly suggests that the single most important key to football safety has been and will always be, the coach. The preparation, the skills, and the awareness of his/her role regarding the ultimate goals of participation are all important in the issue of safety.

An awareness of the following coaching strategies, derived from my 34 years of experience, and from the consensus of several established authors in the field, [28] will lower the probability of player injury.

Football Coaching Safety Strategies

(1)   Understand that your first consideration is to the welfare and education of the student-athlete. This term should really be the "athlete-student." If coaches were taught to carry out this fundamental charge, injuries in athletics would be appreciably lowered. Care and concern for people is the key to safer football. It starts with the coach.

---

[1]Sport safety consultant, serving school districts, athletic associations, recreation departments, camps, insurance companies, and law firms in the area of sport safety. A coach, teacher, and athletic administrator for 34 years, who has served as an expert witness for 27 years. Twelve Narbrook Park, Narberth, PA 19072.

(2)   Understand what society is dictating as the duties of football coaches in terms of safety. Too often coaches are too "tradition oriented," and have a "this is the way my coach taught me" attitude, that they fail to avail themselves of current literature and knowledge. These duties are:

(a)   To condition the player properly at the start of the season to keep good physical conditioning throughout the year. Remember, proper conditioning includes proper rest time to prevent overuse injury,

(b)   to warn the player and his/her parents properly of the potential hazards of the game of football. This must be reinforced throughout the season,

(c)   to offer proper and well-fitting equipment,

(d)   to offer proper and reasonable facilities,

(e)   to supervise the players properly,

(f)   to instruct the players properly, and

(g)   to offer proper medical care.

For more detail concerning the above duties, see Nygaard, Patterson, and van der Smissen [9–11].

In my opinion, safety does not start with the premise of meeting your legal duties; it starts with an attitude of care for people and understanding one's legal duties.

(3)   The playing for a program, practice, or game should include safety considerations. Safety is not a one-time meeting, a one-time speech, or the signing of an informed consent to play form. It is part of every activity.

(4)   A coach is a hazard manager. A coach must:

(a)   recognize a potential hazard,

(b)   remove the hazard,

(c)   if it cannot be removed, cover the hazard, if part of the playing area, and

(d)   if you cannot cover the hazard, remove the participants from the hazard.

(e)   if you cannot remove the participant from the area (there may be no other area), adjust the playing area so the hazard no longer places players in harm's way. This often means making the area smaller, or limiting the activity.

(f)   if you cannot do any of the above, cancel the activity. "Hazard Management" includes the continual instruction and supervision of the staff.

(5)   Maintain records of everything you do. Keep them for at least six years. Records such as informed consent forms, medical examination forms, policies and manuals, injury reports, return to play forms, emergency procedures, maintenance requests, equipment purchases, and practice plans should be kept.

(6)   Equalize competition. Be especially sensitive to size and experience during the early part of the season.

(7)   Seek assistance from administrative sources. We often forget that a major role of the athletic director is to help the coach to help the student athlete. Running a safe program should be a priority. If it is not, there is something wrong. Athletic directors can keep coaches abreast of new equipment, conferences, teaching aids, sports medicine issues, and their legal duties.

(8)   Have a licensed/certified athletic trainer on staff. If the coach is the key to safety, the certified athletic trainer is the insurance. All football programs should have a qualified athletic trainer.

(9)   Create a safety committee that creates and *uses* a safety checklist. Ask a parent, the maintenance department head, the business manager as well as coaches and the athletic trainer to be members of this group. Continual evaluation is a major aspect of any risk management program.

(10)   Read and follow the rules! Stay current with new information and equipment. For example, should high school football programs play by college rules? They should not. They should follow the National High School Rules Book. How many coaches know that the rules define how a tackle is to be executed? They should refer to page 26 of the 1995 rule book. Are coaches aware that the use of the head as a weapon is forbidden not only for the defensive player, but also for the ball carrier and blocker? Watch some football films and you will be surprised at the number of "spearing" used by the offense. Do neck rolls help prevent neck injuries? The literature is unclear.

(11)   Coaches must be able to say "NO!"—No, you can't play until you see a doctor. No, you can't work out in the weight room without a supervisor. No, you can't stay after practice and practice your punting without a coach. No, you're not going back into the game until checked by the doctor!

(12)   Coaches can lower the possibility of injuries by avoiding situations that increase their likelihood [12]. The following are examples of football situations that have either been discussed or listed as part of a legal action against a school and coach. (I have been involved, as a consultant, in each of the situations.)

(a)   taking that last phone call instead of supervising the arriving players,

(b)   giving one coach too many players to supervise,

(c)   letting a player officiate a game because an official did not arrive,

(d)   not properly preparing a team physically. A coach skipped or cut short the warm-up to get into "coaching?"

(e)   playing a student who was previously injured without the approval of the athletic trainer and team physician,

(f)   not having an emergency safety plan,

(g)   permitting players to use poor fitting equipment,

(h)   using correct equipment in an improper manner. A football blocking sled manufacturer was sued because a junior high player was injured while using their sled. The investigation showed that the players, with the approval of the coach, would attempt to "flip over" the seven man sled in order to "get out of doing wind sprints." This inappropriate use of the sled resulted in a leg injured,

(i)   hiring poorly-trained assistants. Hire coaches that know how to teach young people first and the game of football second, and

(j)   using new, but untested strategies or equipment. Remember the movable football blocking dummy that worked on a spring release? The coach released a blocking dummy that moved down a track at various speeds for the waiting player to block it. Unfortunately some players were either not ready or skilled enough to neutralize the force of the traveling dummy. This new piece of equipment, fortunately, disappeared after several major accidents.

(13)   Begin. Get involved. Reread the above and get started. We have offensive coaches, defensive coaches, and specialist coaches. We need safety coaches.

Recommendations

The above discussion suggests several proposals to improve football safety at the scholastic level.

(1)   To establish a national certification standard, I propose that the several youth, state, school, and sport safety organizations already making significant contributions "get together" and begin the process that has been talked about for years. If we "build it, they will come!"

(2)   It is essential to instruct coaches properly on how to teach young people to play the game of football properly.

(3)   Coaches must be encouraged to believe in the stated educational goals of the athletic experience. This is basic, yet it is a major factor in reducing injuries.

(4)   To reconsider the teaching of the tackle. Studies clearly suggest that most injuries occur while in the act of tackling [13–16]. Although while the banning of the helmet as a weapon (the so-called "spearing" rule) in 1976 made a significant difference in serious head and neck injuries, tackling remains a high risk action. Football coaches, officials, and administrators should consider supporting the present and long-standing definition that states, "Tackling is grasping or encircling an opponent with hands or arms" (NCAA, rule 2, p. 25 of 1986). The official high school rules state tackling "is use of hands, arms or body by a defensive player in his attempt to hold a runner or to bring him to the ground" (Art. 8, section 2 of 1992–93). One needs only to watch any level of the game to recognize the many deviations in today's form of tackling. Watch the NFL's popular videos on "great hits," and you will see the glorification of incorrect tackling.

This writer suggests the incorporation of the rugby-type teaching relative to the art of tackling. This is a step-by-step presentation of the elements involved in tackling. Emphasis is on shoulder contact at the upper thigh/torso area, grasping the ball carrier, and using the ball carrier's momentum to bring him to the ground. No true rugby coach would include the "hurt him" philosophy in the skill of tackling. The head is never part of the tackle. The rugby tackle itself, contrary to popular belief, is a different and safer style of tackling. Rugby-style tackling should be taught to our football youth. This is a topic for another paper.

Conclusion

Many factors help to lower the potential of injuries in football for those who play the game. Research, the development of standards, equipment, and facilities are major components of safety. The most important factor, however, is the human factor: the well-trained, administration-supported, vigilant, student-oriented coach.

References

[1]   Kanaby, R., (publisher), "*Official High School Football Rules Book*," National Federation of State High School Associations, Kansas City, KS 1995.
[2]   Adams, S. H., Marlene, J. A. and Bayless, M. A., *Catastrophic Injuries in Sports: Avoidance Strategies*, Benchmark Press, Inc., Indianapolis, 1987.
[3]   Arnold, D. E., "Legal Considerations in the Administration of Public School Physical Education and Athletic Programs," C. C. Thomas, Springfield, 1983.
[4]   Baley, J. A. and David, L. M., "Law and Liability in Athletics," *Physical Education and Recreation*, Allyn and Bacon, Inc., Boston, 1984.
[5]   Borkowski, R. P., *Safety in School Sports and Fitness*, J. W. Walch, Ed., Portland, 1991.
[6]   Dougherty, N. J., "Principles of Safety in Physical Education and Sport," *American Alliance for Health, Physical Education, Recreation, and Dance*, Reston, 1987.
[7]   Koehler, R. W., *Law, Sport Activity and Risk Management*, Stipes Publishing Company, Champaign, IL, 1991.
[8]   Martens, R., *Successful Coaching*, Leisure Press, Champaign, IL, 1990.
[9]   Nagaard, G., *Law for Physical Educators and Coaches*, Brighton Publishing Co, Salt Lake City, 1981.

[*10*] Patterson, A., Esq., "How Athletic Directors and Coaches Can Survive the Lawyer's Game," *Interscholastic Athletic Administration,* Vol. 15, No. 1, 1988, pp. 6–9, and Vol. 15, No. 2, 1988, pp. 6–9.
[*11*] Van Der Smissen, B., *Legal Liability and Risk Management for Public and Private Entities,* Anderson Publishing Co., Cincinnati, 1990.
[*12*] Borkowski, R. P., "Avoiding the Gavel," *Athletic Management,* October/November, 1993, pp. 22–26.
[*13*] Appenzeller, H., Ed., *Sports and Law, Contemporary Issues,* The Michie Company, Charlottesville, 1985.
[*14*] Cunningham, R., "36% of High School Football Players Sidelined by Injury," *National Athletic Trainers' Assoication,* Press Release, 1994.
[*15*] Mueller, F. O., "Tackle Football," *Safety in Team Sports,* American School and Community Safety Association, Washington, DC, 1980.
[*16*] Mueller, F. O. and Dick, S., "Football Fatalities Lowest in 64 Years," *National Federation News,* April, 1995, pp. 4–6.

Bibliography

Appenzeller, H. and Appenzell, T., *Sports and the Courts,* The Michie Company, Charlottesville, 1980.

Appenzeller, H. and Guy, L., *Successful Sport Management,* The Michie Company, Charlottesville, 1985.

Ball, R., "Catastrophic Injury: Why Must It Be?," *The First Aider,* 1985.

Bucher, C. A., *Administration of Physical Education and Athletic Programs,* C. V. Mosby, St. Louis, 1983, p. 559.

Rockett, F. X., "Injuries Involving the Head and Neck: Clinical and Anatomic Aspects," P. F. Vinger and E. F. Hoerner, Eds., *Sport Injuries, The Unthwarted Epidemic,* Boston, Wright, PSG, Inc., 1982.

K. S. Clarke[1]

Football Injuries, Safety Standards, and Insurance Underwriting

REFERENCE: Clarke, K. S., "**Football Injuries, Safety Standards, and Insurance Underwriting,**" *Safety in American Football, ASTM STP 1305,* Earl F. Hoerner, Ed., American Society for Testing and Materials, 1996, pp. 172–175.

ABSTRACT: American football produces injuries, which produce costs, which produce expectations for two types of insurance: accident/medical and liability. Underwriters for insuring carriers rely on "experience" and the interpretation of that experience to determine the "whether" and "how much" of coverage. For accidents and the direct costs experienced, this is a more objective process than for liability. For the latter, the standards against which a defendant would be judged can be objective if available from a standard-promulgating source, or they must be derived from the opinion of an array of experts. ASTM provides a process for capturing expert consensus when it exists.

KEYWORDS: sports injury, football, liability, risk, sports insurance

In whatever sport, continuous awareness of the nature and frequency of the catastrophic injury must be encouraged, not feared, so that contentions of mechanism can be shared for plausibility, implementation, and study, and so that the shared responsibility of all involved, including the participant, can be sorted, understood, and merged for the sake of the participant [1]. This is especially true for football, in which the years have shown both the successes and the lapses in doing those things that do indeed affect the frequency of catastrophic injury. It is also true from another perspective. By dealing faithfully and effectively with the formally catastrophic injury, one can better deal with the less severe, but significant, injury that frequents the sport.

It is a given that football produces a variety of injuries, which produce costs, which in turn produce expectations for insurance. With all the forces at play in a sport like football that utilizes the impact of efficient body contact, the only true solution can be to stop playing. That not being the intent, the reduction of injuries and their costs should be a win, win, win situation for everyone. Between the sport's institutional and equipment providers, participants, and insurers, there should be no adversarial relationships.

However, there can be a huge difference between sincere intentions and actual results when clear standards are not present for reference. When there is no consensus as to the nature and/or extent of an injury problem, or as to the nature and/or extent of a solution to a consensus problem, adversarial positions appear. The implications for insurers differ according to the two basic types of insurance needed.

Insurance Coverages

There are two basic types of sports insurance—medical and liability. Medical insurance, essentially, is for paying, up to the limits of the policy, the actual costs of treatment and

[1]Senior vice president/Risk Analysis, SLE Worldwide Inc., Fort Wayne, IN 48604.

professional care for injuries incurred as an athlete. Liability insurance, essentially, is for paying, up to the limits of the policy, the costs of having hurt someone by negligence—whether in terms of bodily injury, nonphysical personal injury, or loss in property.

Whichever type, the costs of the insurance premium to a sports provider is determined by underwriters, principally from actual experience based on the losses from prior policy periods. Unlike homeowners and auto insurance coverages, sports underwriters do not have the convenience of automatic ratings by factoring in a few variables from years of experience. The few insurers who specialize in sport-related risks may have a developing database that is retrievable and interpretable for this purpose, and are expected to have a feel for what is known as to the nature and extent of the injuries being produced by football, but the final premium is a judgement call that is deemed to be both profitable and marketable.

The better that judgement call, the better the insurer's role in the sport. It does not help the sport either to pay excessive premiums for its necessary coverages, or to have excessive costs relative to premium which would drive the quality insurers away from the vagaries of sports risks. Insurance brokers and agents who arrange for sports coverages have to rely on quality carriers who see the sport as profitable, and these carriers in turn must rely on reinsurers, big money companies, to commit to backing their losses should, by bad luck or bad underwriting, a series of high cost losses be experienced in a short period of time. Within the past decade, we have already seen a period when quality carriers walked away from sports and a nonquality carrier who left its insureds without the funds to pay the costs of the losses for which they had purchased coverage.

It is necessary to differentiate between each of these types of coverage for implications for consensus standards.

Medical Insurance

In sports, medical insurance is typically designed as "Participant Accident Insurance" (P.A.) to spare athletes most of the direct medical costs associated with injury during participation in sport activities. One must read the policy to know all terms and conditions, but typically: coverage involves competitions and supervised practices, with travel to and from competition covered if as a team. Illnesses and pre-existing conditions are excluded. Any relevant insurance already covering the athlete (from work, school, spouse, or parents) would be tapped first. Any combination of deductibles, special concerns, and limits of reimbursement for medical costs can be selected. Limits typically range from $10 000 to $25 000 but can be as high as $100 000 per occurrence.

In addition, a special P.A. coverage—Catastrophic Medical ("Cat Med") Insurance—can be added to a basic P.A. plan for the rare severe permanent injury that brings far more expenses than would be covered by P.A. insurance. Not only does the Cat Med plan provide medical limits of $1,000,000 or higher, it also can provide for guaranteed income and costs of home/auto renovation for wheelchair use that are not included in basic P.A. coverages.

Insurance premiums are investments in the primary purpose of helping the athlete be spared the costs of injuries incurred while participating. The ideal coverage for the athlete and sponsor is a planned merging of basic P.A. and "Cat Med" plans. A plan that uses adequate P.A. insurance for the type of injuries expected in that sport as the deductible for a "Cat Med" plan serves the athlete fully and makes the best use of the sponsor's premium dollar. It also relieves the sponsor's conscience, should a paralyzing accident strike one of its players, by helping the stricken athlete and family face the bills that lie ahead.

The sponsor's participant *liability* insurance may benefit as well when merged with quality P.A. and Cat Med coverage. Often it is when the medical bills exceed coverages that the athlete or family seem to turn to a lawsuit for financial relief. In addition, the continuous review of injury patterns enabled by tracking P.A. claims can lead to improved injury control in that sport and thus to fewer liability as well as P.A. claims.

As for the relevance of standards, medical insurance would of course be influenced by breakthroughs in minimizing certain patterns of injury in football by better equipment, blocking/tackling techniques, officiating, and field management. However, standards for managing the costs of treatment are having much more influence on cost experience and thereby on future premiums than any other consideration. Managed health care with its structured costs is to medical insurance today what helmet standards and rule changes were in the 1970s to liability insurance.

Liability Insurance

While Medical insurance is a form of "no-fault" insurance, Liability insurance is for "at-fault," when the insured is alleged to have been negligent. Different forms of liability insurance exist for the different forms of alleged negligence: "General Liability" for claims from body injury, personal injury (e.g., libel, slander), and/or third party property damage against a corporate entity; "Professional Liability" for the same against a professional person; "Product Liability" for injury caused by the manufacturer of the implicated product; "Directors & Officers Liability" (D&O) for injury caused by the decisions of the individuals who govern the practices of the offending corporate entity; and, "Errors & Omissions Liability" (E&O) for claims against the corporate entity for injury caused by staff error/omission in carrying out the policies of the corporation.

Whichever form of complaint, Negligence is determined by the process of establishing that there had been a duty to protect the injured party from such harm, that a minimum standard of care accompanied that duty, that that standard of care was not provided, and harm resulted directly from that breach in providing the expected standard of care. Moreover, "determination" is made by a panel of "peers" who vote that one of the two teams of experts, plaintiff's and defendant's, is more convincing than the other as to the central question, the applicable standard of care. Consider a football game without points or scoreboard, with the referee asking the crowd at the end of the game to vote which team was a more convincing winner. Such is how our system works, and such is why consensus standards (even if consensus is no standards exist) are so important.

More specifically, it is less the nature of the problem than "the extent of the problem" and "the extent of the solution" that affects the insurer's role in enabling injury-producing sports to remain available in this society. We have little difficulty honoring different professional insights into pathology, etiology, and even epidemiology. It is when that discussion crosses into thresholds for what is *acceptable* as an inherent problem and what is *unacceptable* as preventive action that we begin hearing what *must* instead of what *might* be done about the explained problem. It is then when we most clearly see the intrusion of claims of negligence against liability coverages.

Standards

We have various forms of standards, e.g., the rules of the game; laws and regulations; formal consensus standards; opinions of experts; and information within the promotional materials of the enterprise. Impact testing for helmets, for example, establishes thresholds above which the impact attenuation is not acceptable. Standards-making bodies such as ASTM are in the business of processing such thresholds as consensus standards. It is then up to the sport and others offering programs in which helmets are used to adopt those standards as their's as well.

It is easy then for underwriting to make compliance with a consensus standard a requirement for insurability as well.

It is when the threshold is determined only by a sincere sports safety professional, a product manufacturer, or unilaterally by any interest group that underwriters have problems with what a jury's consensus will be and the consequent premium to keep insurance a profitable business. Another problem is the use of a particular standard for contexts that the standard and its development did not address.

Perhaps there is need for formalization of a standard-promulgating organization to label an issue "consensus of no consensus" until an acceptable threshold is found. We already have it passively, in that no draft of a proposed ASTM standard can be quoted or used in any fashion to intimate consensus. Maybe it is time to classify the issue actively as "without consensus," and/or to use "guidelines" or "working principles" when the measurement of a given threshold is premature.

In the meantime, what we have dealt with in this Symposium and will continue to deal with in future football seasons is best characterized by the verb, "minimizing" instead of "preventing." Sports cannot be made safe, only safer. We can still pursue our common goal, but not create an unnecessary liability via an unattainable or unreasonable expectation.

Reference

[1]   Clarke, K., "Cornerstones for Future Directions in Head/Neck Injury Prevention in Sports," *Proceedings of the Head & Neck Injuries in Sports Symposium,* ASTM, 1994.

Phillip M. Davis[1]

American Football in the Courtroom—Legal Liability Associated with the Game

REFERENCE: Davis, P. M., "**American Football in the Courtroom—Legal Liability Associated with the Game,**" *Safety in American Football, ASTM STP 1305,* Earl F. Hoerner, Ed., American Society for Testing and Materials, 1996, pp. 176–183.

ABSTRACT: This paper reviews the development of the game of football, and its accompanying risk of injury and the various rule changes over time brought about to reduce injuries. The development of litigation related to football injuries is detailed including the potential liability of all associated with the game.

KEYWORDS: Neck injury, NOCSAE, rules, helmet, game film, catastrophic injury, cervical spine, paralysis, spearing, coach, lawsuit, litigation

History

Football is a game of violent contact that inevitably produces injuries. This has been so since Nov. 6, 1869, on a cold, blustery day in New Brunswick, New Jersey, when Rutgers and Princeton played the first intercollegiate football game. Much has changed in the ensuing 125 years. It was initially a game similar to soccer with 25 men on a side and no uniforms. Rules prohibited running or throwing the ball requiring that it be kicked or headed. Scoring was achieved by kicking the ball through the opponent's goal which was 8 yd wide. The first team to kick six field goals won. There was no clock. The field was 120 yd long and 75 yd wide.

Early Injuries

By 1905, crippling injuries and deaths had become of such concern that several colleges, including Columbia, banned the sport because of its brutality. Even President Theodore Roosevelt called for reforms as several states outlawed the sport.

Early Rules and Changes

In 1910, the National Collegiate Athletic Association (NCAA) was formed, in part, to establish rule changes and police the procedures under which members operated their programs. By 1939, head protection was a formal requirement under the rules. By 1951, faceguards became mandatory. In 1976, a pivotal rule prohibiting spearing, ramming, and butt blocking was adopted to stem the tide of rising head and neck (spinal cord) injuries.

Continuing Risk of Injury

Notwithstanding the rule changes and advancements in football, each season, there will be a small, but predictable, number of catastrophic injuries involving permanent quadriplegia as

[1]Partner, Davis and White, 50 Staniford St., Boston, MA 02114.

a result of spinal cord damage or irreversible brain injury. There will also be several deaths of football players. Given the present rules of football, there is nothing that can be done to eradicate completely catastrophic injuries.

Current Technology

The manufacturers of protective equipment are approaching the outer limits of existing technology. The coaching staffs are better educated, more knowledgeable, and more attuned to the athletes' well being and safety than ever before. The trainers, physicians, and other health providers have the benefit of 20 years of intense study of the causes of such catastrophic injuries that occur in football and are prepared to diagnose and treat such injuries promptly and effectively. However, the players are bigger, stronger, and faster than ever before. The energy involved in a full-speed collision between two or more well-conditioned behemoths is enormous. Obviously, no protective equipment can be designed that can be used functionally in the game of football and, yet, protect against all such injuries under these conditions.

Litigation

Unfortunately, in many instances following serious injury or death on the field, the interest of lawyers who envision huge jury awards or large settlements is very predictable. Now, the attorney is just another entrepreneur who disdains investing his time and money in a losing enterprise. The only reason there is not more litigation associated with the game of football is the fact that such suits are expensive and time consuming and far from guaranteed winners. Retention of medical and technical consulting experts by the injured athlete's attorney is an expensive prerequisite and the outcome is frequently unpredictable. In any event, the third inevitability following injuries and attorney interest is litigation against sporting-goods manu-facturers, sporting-goods dealers, high school districts, athletic directors, coaches, trainers, and physicians. The health providers such as the ambulance service, hospital personnel, and physicians may also become involved. Occasionally, the game officials will be named as defendants as will a standard-making body such as the National Operating Committee for the Standards of Athletic Equipment (NOCSAE).

Defense of Helmet Litigation

We have been defending football-related litigation for the past 20 years. During that time, we have handled several hundred claims and lawsuits involving catastrophic brain injury, paralysis, and death. Because history is reputed to repeat itself, it benefits us to look at the cases that have been brought and the theories of recovery that have been set out by plaintiff's counsel. Litigation can arise from the game of football in many situations. In the past, we have defended shoulder pad manufacturers, cleat manufacturers, and have been involved in litigation related to the artificial turf. Likewise, the faceguard has been the focus of some litigation over the years. However, most very serious claims arise from either a catastrophic brain or neck (spinal cord) injury involving suit against the helmet manufacturer and/or coaches, school, and other officials, and we will confine the majority of our analysis of cases to those type of injuries.

When litigation began to proliferate in the 1960s, the claims were generally against the helmet or equipment manufacturer for defective design or manufacturing. During the 1970s, helmet design became more sophisticated (ironically as many stopped making the product) and Riddell and Bike Athletic (now the Air helmet manufactured by Schutt Sports) emerged as the foremost head protection suppliers in the 1980s and 1990s.

As the design and manufacturing processes of the helmet advanced, the plaintiffs' bar shifted their focus to the issue of failure to warn. Warnings were first placed on helmets in 1980 and became required equipment in the mid 80s. As warnings came to be in general use, the plaintiffs' bar again shifted its interest to human factors considerations. Was the helmet too heavy, too light, too big, etc.? Was it fitted properly? Were the correct use and rules taught (i.e., proper blocking and tackling techniques)?

Other Targets of Litigation

As equipment manufacturers began to defend their product more vigorously, attorneys searched for other less legally sophisticated, yet deep-pocket defendants. Most school districts and coaching staffs fall into this category in jurisdictions in which there is no bar of municipal immunity. Hence, in most states, the coach, athletic director, or trainer may well be sued for failure to warn adequately, to instruct adequately, to inform the athlete of the risks of playing, although injured and failing to see to it, that the athlete was provided with a safe environment, including an appropriate playing field, quality equipment, experienced coaches, and available emergency medical assistance.

The reconditioner of football equipment may also be a target defendant because it is his or her purported responsibility to return to the school only with head protection that can remain effective, and meet, or exceed all standards.

Finally, a team physician or coach may be the target of a suit for permitting a player to resume contact when not yet fully recovered from a prior head injury (resulting in the second impact/sudden death phenomena), or from failing to recognize a brain injury promptly (particularly a slow bleeding subdural hematoma), and arrange for immediate medical attention.

Last, the emergency room and other hospital personnel, as well as the ambulance team, may be the target of a lawsuit when the plaintiff's attorney cannot ascertain clearly that there was any evidence of negligence on the part of the equipment manufacturer, coaches, or trainer.

The reader is referred to three game films of incidents that we have defended. Ironically, football is one of the few arenas where the incident is the subject of the litigation, and is frequently recorded for posterity on a game film or video. The film involves three catastrophic neck injuries that occurred in Massachusetts (Williams), Louisiana (Brandt), and Mississippi (Moore). In each instance, the injured player plaintiff lowered his head while attempting a tackle and made helmet-first contact with the ball carrier or another player.

Considerations of Potential Defendants in Catastrophic Injury Cases

The majority of catastrophic football injuries involve damage to the spinal cord with resulting permanent quadriplegia. This injury invariably occurs when the injured player attempts a tackle or, occasionally, as a runner, lowers his head and makes contact with an opposing player with the top or crown of his helmet. The neck is a relatively delicate structure comprised of seven cervical vertebra supported by various ligaments, tendons, cartilage, and muscle. Most severe neck injuries occur when the player lowers his head while making contact, thus straightening the cervical spine that generally is in a slight (lordotic) curve (i.e., axial loading). The straightened spine is caught between the helmeted head that stops upon impact and the weight of the torso that continues forward. The spine buckles usually causing cervical fracture at C4, 5, or 6, and impingement of the spinal cord resulting in permanent paralysis.

The only way this injury can be avoided is for a player always to make contact with his head up. Accidental head-down contact produces a number of these injuries. Occasionally, a well-meaning teammate will move the injured player before the coaches or medical personnel come to his aid. It is imperative to follow proper handling techniques, including leaving the helmet in place until experienced medical technicians are able to take charge. The head, neck, and back should be maintained in alignment.

Manufacturer of Helmet

The manufacturer must meet a design criterion that enables it to produce a functional head protection at an affordable price. Considerations include:

- size (not too large or small);
- allowances for adequate vision and hearing;
- ventilation to prevent heat buildup;
- adjustable fit to accommodate various head shapes and sizes;
- readily repairable or replaceable parts (during game);
- element resistant (sun, rain, cold, snow, and humidity);
- chemical resistant (hair spray, sweat, and ultraviolet rays);
- reconditionable to help control costs;
- paintable;
- proper snug fit and maintain position;
- functional in very hot, very cool weather, or at high altitude;
- weight of the helmet;
- capable of managing energy of multiple contacts;
- capable of managing varying degrees of energy;
- capable of containing adequate warnings and instructions; and
- affordable.

Dealer or Sporting Goods Retailer

The dealer generally has a pass through liability. That is, he may claim back against the manufacturer and receive complete indemnification. Exceptions may include:

(1)   when the dealer makes promises or warranties about the helmet or equipment that are different and greater than those of the manufacturer,

(2)   when the dealer participates in the fitting and misfits a helmet to a player, and

(3)   when the dealer fails to pass on warnings, instructions, or other information with the product or dilutes the warnings in some way by holding the product out to be safer than it is.

School District

(1)   The school district may be responsible for failing to obtain an appropriate permission slip that clearly identifies the nature and extent of the risk, including the possibility of death, so that both player and his parents assume the risk of injury (barring negligence of some other entity) under normal circumstances.

(2)   The school district has an obligation to hire coaches who are skilled and knowledgeable in the game of football, and have the best interest of the players at heart.

(3)   The school district must provide adequate facilities, including an appropriate playing field with sufficient out-of-bounds space, and free of any irregularities in the playing surface that may cause injury.

(4)   The school district, likewise, is responsible for providing adequate equipment and seeing to it that it is regularly maintained or reconditioned.

(5)   The school may be responsible to provide an athletic trainer, an ambulance at games, or even practices, and to have a doctor in attendance at least at games.

(6)   A school, likewise, may be responsible for the overall supervision of the programs to insure that the players' safety needs are reasonably met.

Coaches

The coach's responsibility is somewhat parallel to that of the school but in some instances of a more secondary nature.

(1)   The coach has a principal responsibility to see that every player is properly fitted for his helmet and knows to speak to a coach, trainer, or equipment manager if the helmet is underinflated, too loose or too tight, or has any other problem.

(2)   The coach has a responsibility to teach proper blocking and tackling techniques.

(3)   The coach has a responsibility to show videos or make available other graphic information to players, explaining such techniques and warning of the dangers inherent in the sport if such techniques are not followed.

(4)   The coach has a duty not to send a player back into a game who has experienced a concussion or has a suspected head injury or any other injury that may be exacerbated by further contact.

(5)   The coaches are responsible for knowing and complying with the rules, the National Federation of High School rules or NCAA rules depending on their state rules.

(6)   Many football injuries or deaths are associated with dehydration or heat prostration. The coach should be mindful of this in hot or humid climates, and arrange for adequate water supply and appropriate rest periods.

Athletic Trainer

The athletic trainer is responsible for the proper conditioning of the athlete, for first aid care, for holding the athlete out of any contact in the face of a suspected head injury, and to report and coordinate with the coach as to the proper well being of the athletes.

Team Physician

The team doctor is responsible for emergency medical care on the field, properly diagnosing any suspected head or neck injury, and immediately arranging for appropriate medical care.

EMTs

The emergency medical technicians or ambulance personnel who may be at a game or practice or summoned at the time of an injury are obligated to be familiar with proper handling techniques, first aid, and transportation techniques in the management of the catastrophically brain- or spinal-cord-injured player including the nonremoval of the helmet in suspected neck injuries.

Catastrophic Brain Injuries

Catastrophic brain injuries are frequently of more incipient etiology. Injury may initiate from hard contact that leaves the player momentarily stunned, dazed, or confused. There may be a brief period of unconsciousness and resulting short-term memory loss. However, the player soon appears normal and either does not leave the game or denies any residual effects of the contact. There are between 250 000 and 400 000 documented concussions in football each year. The only surprising fact is that there are not more catastrophic brain injuries. In any event, such an injury can lead to a subdural hematoma, diffuse axonal injury, intercranial cerebral swelling, or edema or the "second impact syndrome or both."

An acute subdural hematoma generally becomes readily apparent. Within minutes of the contact, the player becomes disoriented, nauseated, and loses consciousness. His posturing will become decorticate or decerabate, and usually one pupil will be dilated and fixed. Such a condition mandates immediate surgical intervention or at least hospitalization. The more incipient injury is the subacute or chronic subdural or "slow bleeder." The initial vascular disruption is not sufficient to produce intercranial swelling, and pressure on the brain stem sufficient to produce severe headaches or unconsciousness. The player will continue to participate in contact drills generally without disclosing to the coach that he is experiencing postcontact headaches. Investigation generally demonstrates that the player was complaining to his teammates, friends, girlfriend, and other peers (but not his parents or coaches) of headaches. He is likely to have ingested large quantities of aspirin from the time of his first injury until his collapse. Most players are loath to disclose the presence of such an injury because they know it will keep them on the bench. It's imperative for the coach, trainer, and team physician to monitor any player who has experienced a head or suspected head injury, to exercise caution, and when any doubt arises, to remove the player from the contact, and to secure a complete medical evaluation including CT scans or an MRI. The coach should encourage other players to speak privately to a coach if they become aware that a teammate has headaches because it may save his life.

Perhaps, the more problematic head injury is the second impact syndrome. It is the instance in which the player sustains a slight concussion or apparently insignificant head injury, but returns to play before he is asymptomatic. The brain is now physiologically predisposed to become catastrophically damaged on a second, sometimes relatively inconsequential hit. The autoautonomous centers of the brain regulating blood pressure fail to respond properly permitting more blood to enter the brain than to leave it. This produces vascular engorgement, intercranial swelling, and irreversible brain stem injury, and may produce diffuse brain injury or death or both. We have defended cases involving serious brain injury, and careful investigation almost inevitably discloses a prior injury that was untreated and undisclosed to the coaching staff. It generally happens to a player who is either a team leader or one who lacks the physical gifts of a true athlete, but makes up for his shortcoming with hurtle and vigorous contact to overcome these deficits with determination and a hard-nosed "play injured" attitude.

Coaches Response

The basic problem confronting the football coach is not only his own desire to win, but that of his players, assistant coaches, school, and residents of the town or school district. Although the vast majority of coaches have the safety, well-being, and personal development of their players at heart, it is often difficult to convince players that they must report any head injury, including persistent headaches, dizziness, vision changes, nausea, or other mental disturbance.

Causes of Litigation

Likewise, as game films are studied, any player must be reprimanded or disciplined or both for repeated head-first contact when tackling or carrying the ball. There is absolutely no place in football for the player who persists in head-first contact. It behooves a coach to document the approaches suggested in this paper because the injured player often fails to remember that he was repeatedly taught proper coaching techniques, that he was warned that he could be subject to a catastrophic injury, and that he should report any injury. The majority of lawsuits are brought by players several years after the accident occurs. At the time of the injury, there is usually an outpouring of sympathy by the community that involves fund raisers and contact by both the coaching staff and fellow teammates. However, as the years pass, the players move on to college and other jobs, the insurance provided by the school runs out and the coaching staff either moves on or maintains only sporadic contact. The injured player is left as a financial and physical burden to his family and often litigation appears the only way to solve this dilemma partially. Often the family is bitter at the end result and searches for a scapegoat.

The legal profession is not without its share of blame for the commencement of groundless lawsuits because juries are naturally sympathetic towards a quadriplegic or severely brain-injured youngster. Indeed, virtually every lawsuit resulting in a plaintiff's verdict against a school, coaches, or helmet manufacturer has been produced by sympathy more so than evidence of neglect or defect. The following is a bibliography of football litigation cases that may prove of interest to members of the audience. They are the court's reports following actual lawsuits involving catastrophically injured young men while playing football.

Bibliography of Football Litigation Cases

Dente v. Riddell, 664 F.2d 1 (1981).
Carrier v. Riddell, Inc., 721 F.2d 867 (1983).
Lister v. Bill Kelley Athletic, Inc., 137 Ill. App. 3rd 829, 485 N.E. 2d 483 (Ill. App. Dec. 672 1985).
Struder v. Riddell Co., ——— Ct of Appeals of Tennessee, April 27, 1984.
Gentile v. MacGregor Manufacturing Company, 201 N.J. Super. 612, 493 A.2d 647 (1985).
Fiske v. MacGregor, 464 A.2d 7190 (R.I. 1983).
Rawlings Sporting Goods Co. v. Daniels, 619 S.W. 2d 435 (Tex. Civ. App. 1981).
Boulet v. Brunswick Corp., 107 Mich App. 309 N.W. 2d 680 (1981).
Byrns v. Riddell, 113 Ariz. 264, 550 P.2d 1065 (1976).
Galindo v. Riddell, Inc., 107 Ill. App. 3d 139, Ill. App. 437 N.E. 2d 276 (1982).
Lynch v. Riddell, Inc., 35 Fed Rules Serv. 2d 185 (1982).
Thomas v. Chicago Board of Education, 77 Ill. 2d 165 (1979).
Peterson v. Multnomah County School District No. 1, 68 Or. App. 81, 668 P.2d 385 (1983).
Little v. Bay View Area Red Cats, Inc., 103 Wis, 2d 690, 309 N.W. 2d 889 (1981).
Knight v. Jewett, 3 Cal.4th 296, 11 Cal Rptr.2d 2 (1992).
Jemaa v. MacGregor Athletic Products, 151 Mich. App. 273, 390 N.W.2d 180 (1985).
Eldridge v. Riddell, 626 So.2d 232 (1993).
Whipple v. Salvation Army, 261 Or. 453, 495 P.2d 739 (1971).
Hackbart v. Cincinnati Bengals, 601 F.2d 516 (1979).
Laiche v. Kohen, 621 So.2d 1162 (1993).
Kabella v. Bouschelle, 100 N.M. 461, 672 P.2d 290 (1983).
Hale v. Davies, 86 Ga.App. 126, 70 S.E. 923 (1952).
Matute v. Carson Long Institute, 160 F.Supp. 827 (1958).
Parks v. Atlanta Public School System Board of Education, 168 Ga.App. 572, 309 S.E.2d 645 (1983).
Ward v. Community Unit School District Co., 213 Ill.App.3d 1008, 572 N.E.2d 986, 157 Ill.Dec.522 (1991).
Williams v. Board of Education of the City of Chicago, 222 Ill.App.3d 559, 584 N.E.2d 257, 165 Ill.Dec. 78 (1991).
Hemphill v. Sayers, 552 F.Supp. 685 (1982).

Wissell v. Ohio High School Athletic Association, 78 Ohio App.3d 529, 605 N.E.2d 458 (1992).

Leahy v. School Board of Hernando County, 450 So.2d 883 (1984).

Arnold v. Riddell, 1194 WL 246543 (D.Kan. April 5, 1994).

Austria v. Bike Athletic Co., 107 Or.App. 57, 810 P.2d 1312 (1991).

Rutter v. Northeastern Beaver County School District, 283 Pa.Super. 155, 423 A.2d 1035 (1980).

Gerrity v. Beaty, 37 N.E.2d 47, 373 N.E.2d 1323, 15 III.Dec. 639 (1978).

Vendrell v. School District No. 26C Malheur County, 233 Or. 1, 376 P.2d 406 (1962).

Lowe v. Texas Tech University, 540 S.W.2d 297 (1976).

Curtis v. State of Ohio, Ohio State University, 29 Ohio App.3d 297, 504 N.E.2d 1222 (1986).

Thomas v. Chicago Board of Education, 60 III.App.3d 729, 377 N.E.2d 55, 17 III.Dec 865 (1979).

Sullins v. City of Shreveport, 229 So.2d 390 (1970).

Brandt v. Bike Athletic Company; LA Court of Appeals, 4th Cir. No. 93-CA-1416 c/w 93-CA-0457.

Miller v. Bike Athletic Company; Crt. of Appeals, Belmont County, Ohio, 7th Dist., No. 94-B-52.

Mark S. Granger[1]

Safety in Football—Risk Avoidance and Risk Management: An Attorney's Perspective

REFERENCE: Granger, M. S., "**Safety in Football—Risk Avoidance and Risk Management: An Attorney's Perspective,**" *Safety in American Football, ASTM STP 1305,* Earl F. Hoerner, Ed., American Society for Testing and Materials, 1996, pp. 184–188.

ABSTRACT: The litigation explosion in this country and the ever increasing refusal to accept personal responsibility for ones' own actions has resulted in an increased number of law suits in the sports arena. In addition to manufacturers of football equipment, schools, coaches, and leagues are now being sued. Everyone involved with the sport is exposed. Reduction of injury potential and severity is both good practice and good management in this litigation prone era. The paper discusses ways to reduce injuries and exposure including: better coaching, comprehensive reviews of facilities and programs, proper training of coaches and staff, better and stricter officiating, and proper protective gear, and warnings and instructions. The need for proper and consumer oriented information on the risk of a particular sport to the athlete and his or her family is also stressed. Finally, the role of the technical community in reporting on and reducing sports injuries is analyzed.

KEYWORDS: risk, safety, legal issues, litigation, misuse, products liability, leagues, schools, coaches, coaching, training, facilities, officiating, protective gear, football

It is perhaps a sad commentary on our times when a lawyer needs to make a presentation to a group concentrating on making sports safer. Yet, for reasons set forth in this presentation, it is foolish for anyone in attendance or reviewing the materials from this symposium to avoid a review of the serious legal issues facing football at all levels of play. If a school or coach thinks that legal issues only relate to the manufacturers of equipment, then they are certainly in for a surprise.

A "Risk Free" Society

We live in a society that increasingly refuses to accept risk and personal responsibility in any form. Although this began in the product liability era of the 1970s and 1980s, it now has entwined itself in the very fabric of American life. There is no such thing anymore as an accident, every injury must have a cause and someone to blame. People, including athletes, are no longer willing to admit that they made an error in judgment or were the victims of bad luck. If there is an injury, they are looking for someone to blame, and that someone could be a town, a school, an athletic facility, or a company.

Given this premise, it is therefore probably no surprise that in the event of serious injury in football, and perhaps even in the case of minor injuries, someone is going to be sued. A

[1]Esquire, 250 Summer St., Boston, MA 02210-1181.

plaintiff's lawyer is going to ask a jury to forget that this was a sport and instead insist that his client was blameless for the accident and, therefore, someone should pay. There are a variety of potential defendants available for attack by the plaintiff lawyer. In nearly 18 years of defending companies, towns, and facilities, I have always been struck with plaintiff's counsel's resourcefulness, ability to dig hard for the "deep pocket," and to find an alleged expert who will say anything to put together a case. In such an atmosphere, one has to be ready. Risk avoidance and risk management not only can reduce the chances of being sued, they can also substantially reduce the exposure if a person, town, or company is sued, and enhance their chance of winning. Most importantly, however, they can also result in safer football with fewer injuries.

The Legal Background

The development of products liability law over the past three decades has had a profound impact on sports. Although originally applied to traditional consumer goods such as automobiles, the doctrine of product liability has spread to all aspects of life. Sports is no exception.

Manufacturers are now responsible for product design that takes into account both foreseeable use of those products and foreseeable *misuse* of the products. Products must be reasonably safe for their foreseeable use and misuses. There is a continuing duty to remain informed of the product experience in the market place. How people use a product and the problems they have with it are critical to proper manufacture.

Products must warn about hidden dangers. Although open and obvious dangers need not be warned against, often the burden falls on the manufacturer to show that the danger was open and obvious to the consumer.

The extension of these principles to sports is obvious for manufacturers. It is tougher to see how it applies to coaches, leagues, and schools. Note that the basic principles established in product liability are now being applied to judge the conduct of schools, leagues, and coaches. The technical community also has increased responsibility, for the standards that they establish will set a baseline for behavior expected in the world of sports. It is critical that technical dimensions also include a realization that these dimensions can have critical impact on sports rules, equipment, and on life.

Who Can Be Sued? Virtually Everyone!

So why should anyone reading this article care? Assume that the reader is a coach in a town league, a school, or league administrator, or a teacher at a private not-for-profit high school who is picking up a few dollars by coaching. The answer is that under evolving state law in many jurisdictions, a coach or league administrator can be liable for an athlete's injuries. The states have been slowly chipping away at sovereign immunity and have also removed the ceilings on recovery in many states. Public employees may be personally liable as may the employees and officers of charitable organizations. In Massachusetts, for example, even though there is a limitation on recovery against a not-for-profit organization, there is no limitation on suits against employees of the school or its officers. Real exposure exists for boards of directors and coaches. The athletic facility that does not have modern equipment or accidentally creates a dangerous situation can also be a target. Finally, league officials can be sued if they do not enforce rules designed primarily for safety and an injury results. Manufacturers continue to be a target, more on that below.

In short, it is not just the manufacturers that have to react and take action, it is schools, athletic programs, clubs, coaches, competition officials and league officials. The goal of this presentation is to help schools, town programs, teams, coaches, officials, and manufacturers avoid or greatly reduce their exposure to personal injury claims for athletic injuries.

Preventing Injuries and Reducing Liabilities

There are several ways in which injuries and liability exposures can be reduced:

Proper Coaching

Critical injuries are far more prevalent in school sports than they are in professional sports. One reason for that is more consistent training and emphasis on injury prevention on the field in professional sports. Many injuries take place during plays in which one or more players are and have been violating the rules of the game. Back-checking a hockey player into the boards and spearing and head butting in football are good examples. Coaches must teach good, safe play and *emphasize the importance of the potential consequences of failing to follow coaches's advice.* Players should be informed that head butting or spearing can result in paralysis, brain injury, or death. Schools should insist that their coaches are properly educated on proper and safe techniques. They must provide these resources to their coaches. Use should be made of videos and other materials generally available. Many injuries occur from lack of requisite skills. Coaches must teach fundamental skills of blocking, tackling, and falling well *and* the reasons for those skills.

A Comprehensive Review of All Facilities and Programs

Schools and leagues must hire the appropriate coaches. These coaches must attend meetings on their sport. Access to an outside expert in sports safety and an attorney with sports litigation experience should be obtained. Programs in other schools should be observed and attempts made to determine if there are any standards (ASTM or otherwise) which apply. Consultation with an attorney may be an affirmative defense to negligence claims against a school and league. Staying on top of safety programs is critical for good management of exposure. Schools and leagues should examine their facilities for "hidden" dangers such as unpadded obstructions, poor or damaged running surfaces, and improper clearances around playing zones. All facilities should have an emergency plan in effect to help reduce the impact of an athlete's injury. Facilities should also document and collect information on injuries to look for patterns or repeat injuries. Steps must be taken to modify or provide greater warnings and instructions at facilities.

Coaches and Staff Must Be Properly Trained

Programs should confirm that their coaches and staffs are fully trained with respect to safety within their respective sports. They should attend seminars and other programs (such as this ASTM conference) to be more "injury aware." It is amazing how many coaches know nothing about preventing injuries or how adherence to the rules and proper player education can reduce risk. Training must also take place in first aid and immediate care to prevent injury enhancement and to promote awareness of injury prevention. Trainers and coaches should receive the most up-to-date conditioning information which is often available in seminars. Efforts should be made to obtain training films from manufacturers. We live in a visually oriented society. The best way to reach student athletes on safety issues is through video. Every athletic program should develop *and use* a training and safety video library. An excellent example is the CAPS Program sponsored by the Sporting Goods Manufacturer's Association. In addition to providing videos, this group provides speakers for making presentations to coaches.

Schools and leagues should seek input from medical professionals who are experts in the sports medicine fields. Colleges and universities are now offering sports medicine courses which would provide excellent resources to coaches and leagues.

Better and Stricter Officiating

Players and coaches generally believe that game rules are designed for fair play. It is important to note that another reason for rules and enforcement of penalties for infractions is for safety. Many rules such as clipping, spearing, facemasking, etc in football are safety related. Coaches, players, and officials should be aware of this. Leagues should take substantial steps to enforce rules and emphasize that the rules are also meant for safety. The consequences of violating the rules (such as serious personal injury, a career-ending permanent condition or worse) should be emphasized.

Proper Protective Gear, Warnings, and Instructions

Getting the proper gear, and making sure it is used, fitted, and maintained properly is essential to safe football. In doing this, one has to look at the whole product, including the warnings and instructions that come with it, and the probable, foreseeable misuses of the product. Manufacturers should conduct a comprehensive analysis of their products' safety aspects. An ergonomic specialist and consultants on design, warnings, and instructions should be considered. Often an experienced attorney, particularly one who has had handled cases involving sports injury, can be of major assistance. Both the product and all writings accompanying it and affixed to it must be considered. The risk to manufacturers of failing to do the above is substantial exposure in litigation and the serious costs of defending an action.

Obviously standards for industry must be followed by manufacturers, and efforts should be made and documented to show that these standards are being reviewed in the light of injury experience. Plaintiffs' counsel are increasingly looking at research and development budgets and personnel assignments to try to show that a manufacturer is not dedicating the needed resources to building a safer product. Manufacturers must demonstrate a willingness to go forward on monitoring the use to which their products are put and the nature of the injuries resulting from accidents.

Schools should conduct a complete review and analysis of all protective gear. A consultant and an attorney can be of substantial help in reviewing warnings and instructions provided with the products. The coach should not do this alone as warnings may be inadequate, or there may be confusion between league requirements and the manufacturer's materials.

Reconditioning programs should be carefully examined, and the manufacturers consulted as to whether their equipment can be reconditioned. Reconditioning often results in the removal of all warning labels and instructions from equipment. It can, in some cases, also result in damage to the protective gear. Proper maintenance is the school's responsibility. Only a reputable reconditioner should be used who will stand behind its work. Substantial insurance should be required for all reconditioners.

Information on Safety and Risk Must Be Communicated

Schools and athletic programs have a responsibility to communicate safety rules and risk factors repeatedly to athletes, coaches, and parents. Athletes must understand the risks, and that understanding must be documented. Signing a release form at the beginning of the season is not enough. Coaches need to emphasize safety in practice, and parents need to be informed and updated over the course of the season. Communications on safety should be documented, check lists of documents should be distributed, films must be shown, and lectures given. These methods and their documentation are critical in litigation avoidance and management. The requirement of filling out documentation also serves as a reminder to coaches, administrators, and league officials that safety instruction is a critical part of any athletic program. Again, the risks associated with failure to follow these rules should be strongly emphasized to all. Limitations of the protective gear must also be clearly presented to the athletes. No one should be relying on his or her equipment to prevent all injuries.

The Technical Community Has a Responsibility Too

Members of technical organizations (such as ASTM) have a responsibility to gather information about sports injuries and to look to new ways to avoid or minimize them. More exacting performance standards or better warnings and instructions may be called for based on injuries experienced. The scientific community can help by providing a balanced, intelligent response to injuries in sports.

Conclusion

Safety in sports such as football is no accident. In our society, entities involved at all levels of sport must participate in risk avoidance and risk management. In addition to reducing the chance of litigation involving manufacturers, leagues, schools, or coaches, it can also have the benefit of truly making football safer.

Author Index

Subject Index

A

Abrasiveness, synthetic turf, 103
Anthropometric test devices, 60
Artificial turf, *see* Synthetic turf
ASTM F 355, 123
ASTM F 1551, 103
AstroTurf, field performance over 30 years, 123
Athletic equipment
  certification, 89
  helmet fitting errors, 83
Athletic fields, *see* Football fields

B

Biostatistics, youth football, 21

C

Catastrophic injury, transient quadriplegia, 53
Certification, protective equipment, 89
Cervical spinal cord
  anthropometric test devices, 60
  injuries, 42
  neck protection, 75
  stenosis, 53
Cervical test device, improved, 60
Chinstrap, helmet fitting errors, 83
Coaching
  education, 3
  legal issues, 184
  safety orientation and training skills program, 21, 167
Compliance, protective equipment certification, 89
Compression resistance, synthetic turf, 103
Computed tomography, spinal stenosis, 53
Concussion, management, 35
Conditioning, 167
Contusion, 35
Creeping red fescue, 145
Crumb rubber, turfgrass, 132
Cutting height, turfgrass, 145

D

Dimensions, of facilities, injury prevention, 97
Dissemination, injury prevention information, 3
Dynamic bases, envelope system, 114

E

Envelope system, 114
Epidemiology, youth football, 21
Equipment, safety and, 167
Expert witness, 167

F

Facilities
  dimensions, 97
  legal issues, 184
  safety and, 167
Fall football, NCAA Injury Surveillance System, 9
Fertility, turfgrass, 132
Finite element analysis, anthropometric test devices, 60
Fitting errors, helmets, 83
Flammability, synthetic turf, 103
Football facilities, safety guidelines, 97
Football fields
  enhancing participant safety, turfgrass, 156
  safety guidelines, 97
  traction measurement, 145
  turfgrass, 132

G

G_{max} testing, 123
Grab tear, synthetic turf, 103

H

Head injuries, 35
Helmet, fitting errors, 83

I

Impact absorption, *see* Shock absorbency
Injury
  catastrophic, 42
  comparison of collegiate fall and spring football, 9
  criteria, anthropometric test devices, 60
  helmet fitting errors and, 83
  insurance underwriting, 172
  surface hardness, turfgrass, 156
  youth football, 21
Injury prevention
  barriers to, 3

191